Robin Temple has studied and worked with alternative approaches to health and healing for many years. He currently runs courses for dyslexic children and their parents both in Europe and the United States.

'Your Child' series

A series of books containing easy-to-follow, practical advice for the parents of children with a variety of illnesses or conditions.

Each book provides a clear overview of the situation, explaining essential information about the illness or condition and outlining the practical steps parents and carers can take to help understand, support and care for their child, the rest of the family as well as themselves. Guiding parents through the conventional, the complementary and the alternative approaches available, these books cater for children of all ages, ranging from babies to teenagers, and enable the whole family to move forward in a positive way.

Books in the series:

Asthma, Erika Harvey
Bullying, Jenny Alexander
Dyslexia, Robin Temple
Epilepsy, Fiona Marshall
Headaches & Migraine, Maggie Jones

Your Child

DYSLEXIA

*Practical and easy-to-follow
advice for parents*

ROBIN TEMPLE

ISBN 1-84333-046-6

A catalogue record for this book is available
from the British Library

First published in 2002 by
Vega
64 Brewery Road
London, N7 9NT

A member of **Chrysalis** Books plc

Visit our website at www.chrysalisbooks.co.uk

Printed in Great Britain
by CPD, Wales

This book is dedicated to my wife Siegerdina,
and to my mother Audrey and father Merfyn,
for their unconditional love

and to my very good friends
Ron and Alice Davis
for their inspiration and warmth
and passion to help dyslexics everywhere in the world

Contents

Acknowledgements

I would like to acknowledge the help and support of the following people in writing this book:

Grace Cheetham of Element Books Ltd, for her support and without whom this book would never have happened;

Jane Clitheroe, my dear sister, for her untiring help with the editing and her home cooking;

my colleagues in the Davis Dyslexia Association: Ron and Alice Davis, Sharon Pfeiffer and Abigail Marshall at Davis Dyslexia Association International for their useful feedback and advice; Lin Seward in England, Bonny Beuret in Switzerland and Olga Zambrano in Mexico for their input as mothers of dyslexic children, for their good advice for parents and for their enthusiasm;

all the many dyslexic children and adults I have met and talked to and counselled, for their resourcefulness in the face of their difficulties and for helping me to understand their dyslexia better.

Introduction

When James came to do a Davis Dyslexia Correction Programme he was nine years old, hated school and would cry every morning before leaving home. His worst problem was his handwriting. It was so bad he did not want to write anything. He was so frustrated with not being able to write that he suffered severe cramp in his hand and arm, right up the shoulder. Whenever he was asked to do some writing he was very good at diverting attention onto something else to avoid having to write. In fact James was so depressed and down that whenever he was asked to try and do something his standard reply was always, 'Oh, no! Forget it! I can't do that!' He enjoys going to school now and he writes well and has no trouble with his hand or arm getting stiff.

Michael was 10 when he did a week's programme at a Davis centre. He had come because his parents were at their wit's end about what to do with him. He was far behind at school with his reading and in other subjects and was uncontrollable at home. He was the sort of child who always wanted to be in control. If he was asked to do one thing, he would do the opposite. The counsellor who was working with Michael came into the counselling room one day with a box of clay for the Symbol Mastery (see pages 118–21) and said cheerfully 'We must be careful not to get the clay on the carpet because it is very difficult to get off.' Two minutes later Michael was jumping up and down on the upturned box of clay on the carpet in triumph. It got so difficult with Michael that at one point it seemed as though he would not be able to complete the full five days of the programme. But he did.

His parents soon began to notice all sorts of changes. Michael had hated writing but suddenly he was writing notes to his mother telling her when he was going to be back from school. And he never used to be on time for anything but was now actually arriving in time for supper.

What was best of all for Michael's parents was that they could finally have a normal conversation with him. He could sit quietly and listen, something that he had never been able to do before.

And to add to everything else, in the last two years he has caught up completely with his school work and is now able to keep up with his friends.

Something profound happened in the lives of both these boys and in the lives of their parents and brothers and sisters. The symptoms of dyslexia that had made their lives a misery had disappeared leaving happy, creative and delightful children.

This book is about a new way of understanding and treating dyslexia that allowed these changes to happen for Michael and James. These two boys are in no way special or unique cases. Thousands of children and adults have been able to leave behind disabilities in learning and living that were troubling them and their families. Michael and James perhaps had symptoms that were more extreme than those your child may be suffering. So the changes that occurred for them seem more dramatic. But for the parents of both these boys the dramatic changes were not the most important thing. Obviously it makes a huge difference that Michael and James can now go to school happily and freely, but what their parents were most grateful for was that they had found the sons they always knew were there somewhere.

Nothing essentially had been changed in their children. What was different was that these boys were now able to remove the interference and obstructions that had previously stopped them from learning. This happened slowly over time. Little by little the boys grew in confidence as they explored how to use what they had been taught about their own dyslexia.

So what is this new understanding of dyslexia that can make such differences possible?

Note: 'He' and 'she' have been used to describe your child in alternate chapters to avoid the more cumbersome 'he or she'.

1

What is Dyslexia?

■ A new understanding

For the last 100 years, since the word dyslexia first started being used for a particular form of brain damage that affected the ability to read, we have been stuck with just one point of view about what makes it so difficult for some children to learn.

The common assumption today is that if children have difficulties with such things as reading, spelling, understanding verbal instructions, and organizing thoughts, and if they do such things as reverse letters and numbers, they have a form of dyslexia. This condition of dyslexia is used to explain the difficulties these children have in learning at school and in coping with life.

It is also assumed that the symptoms of dyslexia are caused by some malformation or malfunction of the brain. Many theories exist about why the dyslexic child's brain is not working normally. But no one definite conclusion has been reached about the cause of dyslexia. What everyone can agree with is that it is very difficult and sometimes impossible to help a child with dyslexia. It is also generally accepted that dyslexia is not curable, but it is something that a child will have to learn to live with for the rest of his or her life.

There are many ways being offered today to help a dyslexic person to cope with and compensate for particular difficulties with learning, but the idea that a child's dyslexic symptoms can be 100 per cent corrected is completely new and foreign to almost everyone working in this field. Happily for all dyslexic children and their parents and teachers, the idea that dyslexia can be simply, effectively and permanently corrected does now exist. In fact, dyslexia correction not only exists as an idea but is actually the personal experience of thousands of former sufferers.

Any proposal that contradicts the generally accepted theories and understanding about any subject must be tested and proven before becoming fully accepted and a part of our thinking. This process is now taking place in the field of dyslexia.

■ The 'dyslexia' label

About 15 years ago, Ronald Davis, an engineer and sculptor, discovered something about his own dyslexia that did not fit the label for dyslexia he had been given by his doctor. He noticed that the dyslexia which he had been *told* he had, caused by brain damage, did not fit with the dyslexia which he *saw* that he had.

One day while at work on a sculpture, he observed his own dyslexic symptoms changing before his eyes. What he saw did not match the label that he had been given. He had always been told that 'having dyslexia = having brain damage'. Like many dyslexics, Ron was very curious. The mismatch between his own experience of dyslexia and the explanation that he had been given led him to become a researcher in the field of learning disabilities. What he discovered has completely changed the way we understand dyslexia.

■ Something more?

On the whole most parents of dyslexic children feel somewhat dissatisfied with the way their child's dyslexia is explained to them. Parents who come to the Davis Dyslexic Correction Centre with their children often express the feeling that the dyslexia tests and reports they have had leave something out.

The tests state only what is wrong with their child and do not mention anything that is right. These parents do not experience their child as dumb, lazy or incapable. They see a child who has difficulties in some areas but in others is very talented. 'There must be more to it!' they say.

This book will confirm that there is, indeed, 'something more' that can help to make sense of your child's dyslexia.

■ A change of meaning

The word dyslexia, as a label, was invented more than 100 years ago to identify a particular set of symptoms caused by brain damage in adults.

We all know what happens when a label gets attached to something. Because we are in such a hurry most of the time, with so many things to think about, we get in the habit of just looking at labels and not at what they are attached to. We can end up not understanding what is going on. Although we may be using all the right labels, what they are being applied to may have changed without us realizing. Consequently, our understanding will not fit with what is really there.

This is what has happened in the world of dyslexia over the years. 'Dyslexia' originally meant difficulties with reading caused by damage to the brain in *adults* – an accurate, simple and clear label. But then the label 'dyslexic' started to be applied to *children* who had difficulty reading. Whenever you apply a label the meanings attached to that label come with it. The meaning attached to 'dyslexia' is brain damage or malfunction. The label 'dyslexia' was saying the children could not read because they had brain damage. Even though there was no obvious history of brain damage in these children the label said it must be there because the symptoms fitted the label. Because brain damage is very hard to see and measure and it was doctors who were involved in giving the label, no one else felt able or willing to challenge what they were saying.

It has now become clear that most children with reading

difficulties do not have brain malfunctions. There is another reason why they have dyslexia – and this is what Ron Davis discovered. He managed to peel off his own label of dyslexia. He looked underneath what he had been told to see. He found his reading problems were not the result of his brain working incorrectly.

Over the years people have tried to apply the label dyslexia to more and more symptoms. It has now got to the point where some people are even recommending throwing the word dyslexia away altogether, because it has been stretched so wide that it has lost much of its usefulness as a label.

What Ron Davis set out to do, with a team of researchers, was to find a label that was large enough to fit all the many different symptoms that he found in the dyslexics who came to see him at his Reading Research Council centre. Fortunately for all of us he succeeded. It took three years and a great deal of trial and error, but eventually the research team were able to create a clear picture of what causes learning disabilities.

More and more dyslexics are finding out about this new way of understanding dyslexia. They are very happy, and relieved, that finally someone is talking about dyslexia in a way they can relate to.

■ The two models of dyslexia

There are currently two different understandings of dyslexia available. The model of dyslexia laid down more than 100 years ago, based on the assumption that symptoms are caused by some malformation or malfunction in the brain, has been the accepted way of looking at dyslexia up until the present day. I have called this the Orthodox Model and it is discussed in the following chapter. The new approach to dyslexia developed by Ron Davis over the last 15 years I have called the Davis Model, and this is covered in Chapter 3.

2

The Orthodox Model

■ DEFINITIONS AND THEORIES

■ Early definitions of dyslexia

The word dyslexia was introduced in 1887 by Dr Rudolf Berlin. It was then seen as something that developed rather than something one was born with. He suggested that the inability to read was due to 'cerebral disease' rather than brain injury. Dr J Hinshelwood made a further suggestion that dyslexia came from 'underdevelopment of the angular gyrus', and Dr Samuel Orton in the United States went even further to suggest that dyslexia was a developmental problem combined with environmental factors and was not entirely congenital or passed down from parents to children.

The words you are most likely to hear in connection with dyslexia – apart from the very general terms 'learning disabilities' or 'learning difficulties' that are often used instead of 'dyslexia' – are 'aphasia' and 'word blindness'.

Aphasia

This was the very first word to be used in connection with dyslexia, which was originally defined as a form of aphasia. The technical definition of aphasia is 'loss or impairment of the ability to use or comprehend words due to an injury of the brain'. There are actually four kinds of aphasia:

- sensory aphasia – difficulty understanding spoken language
- motor aphasia – difficulty expressing thoughts through speech
- alexia – difficulty reading
- agraphia – difficulty writing

When dyslexia was introduced as a term it was generally classified under aphasia as a form of alexia.

Word blindness

This term had been introduced in 1877 by Adolph Kussmaul. Although word blindness was thought to be caused by brain injury, the words were also used in connection with patients whose capacities for sight, speech and intelligence were intact but who were not able to recognize words they already knew. The part of the brain responsible for word blindness was proposed as the 'angular gyrus', the part of the brain responsible for speech.

In 1896 Dr W Pringle Morgan in England reported the first case of congenital word blindness in a child.

▧ Another possible 'cause'

The problems of dyslexia obviously existed before scientists and doctors described it in their patients. But it was because of forces outside the world of science and medicine that dyslexia became more than an obscure condition written about in medical journals.

Around the turn of the century the United States and many countries in Europe began to adopt a policy of 'universal literacy'. It was decided by governments that all children should be taught to read and that it was valuable to have all members of society literate. Until this decision was made, non-readers had not been considered a problem. When universal literacy became the new norm it inevitably created a new category of citizens – those who were unable to read or who had great difficulty reading and with school work. These people came to be considered as somehow less than normal. To put it in another way, the norms of the non-dyslexic world were adopted as universal norms. Those who found it uncomfortable to operate in the non-dyslexic world were inevitably discriminated against.

The education system was designed around the non-dyslexic norms. For the few who could not function easily in this system the labels of dyslexia and learning disabled were conveniently at hand.

Since these very early attempts to attribute a cause to the symptoms of dyslexia, much research has been done to test and verify the different hypotheses. Until now, no conclusive proof has been produced.

■ Current research

Present research in dyslexia is focused on four key areas:

1 *Proving that the brain structure of dyslexics is different from that of non-dyslexics.* Various parts of the brain structure are being studied to see if significant differences can be found between dyslexics and other people. If differences are found, it must then be determined whether they are the *cause* or the *result* of dyslexia.

2 *Finding a gene that causes dyslexia.* If such a gene is found, it will be possible to predict that a child will have learning difficulties. Several research laboratories claim to have found the gene that causes dyslexia, but unfortunately each one claims a different gene is responsible.

3 *Comparing the accuracy of different models for explaining dyslexia.* This research covers the various ways of treating learning disabled children. Sets of data are collected from tests based on different models of how dyslexia works. They are then compared to ascertain the effectiveness of each model and which is the most accurate. The difficulty with this sort of research is that it

is very difficult to find a common standard on which to judge different forms of treatment.

4 *Explaining how dyslexics differ from non-dyslexics in processing information in the brain.* Many theories and models presently exist to explain the complex processes that go on when a child is reading. No common agreement can be reached about which parts of the process are at fault. And it is possible that the part of the process at fault will not be the same in all dyslexic children, so there could be many reasons for the same symptoms.

▓ The link between causes and symptoms

The link between the symptoms of dyslexia and the possible causes is very difficult to prove. Each dyslexic child has a different set of symptoms which could derive from any combination of causes. All that can usefully be said about the link is that:

- the symptoms are descriptions of some interference in the way information is processed and reproduced in a child
- where, when and how that interference happens can sometimes be described, and there is sufficient variation to suggest that more than one cause may be operating
- not enough is yet known about the complex processes involved in receiving, processing and producing information to be able to describe any cause accurately

▓ TESTING

▓ Planning

If you decide to have your child tested for dyslexia it is best to begin by making a plan. As with any plan, this involves two steps:

1 Taking stock – knowing where you and your child are right now.

2 Deciding what you want to achieve – knowing where you and your child want to get to and finding the direction and steps to get there.

Taking stock

The following information/documents will help you to gain a clear picture of your child's present situation.

- the age of your child
- the symptoms you can observe in your child
- reports from school (where available) of your child's performance
- (for older children) a history of your child's school career
- any changes in family circumstances
- details and results of any tests carried out specifically for dyslexia
- details and results of any other medical or educational tests
- details and results of any treatments that your child may have had or be having for dyslexia or any other condition

Deciding what you want to achieve

This will be based on the picture of your childs present situation gained from the above list and what you can find out about testing and treatments for your child.

1 Arrange for your child to be tested to determine as far as possible the extent of the disability – both the areas which are affected and the degree to which the disability affects those areas.
2 Based on results of these tests research what treatments for dyslexia are available to your child. Consider the following factors:

- prognosis for correction of disability
- any feelings that your child has about the treatments
- cost of treatments, including both how much time and money will need to be committed

- credentials of persons offering treatments
- practicality of fitting any treatment in with child's other commitments
- effect this treatment programme will have on you as parents and other members of the family

3 Explain to your child what is happening and what your plans are for him. Discuss these plans in such a way that your child can feel included. Choose a treatment that your child also feels positive and cooperative about. Avoid imposing any course of treatment on an unwilling child.

◼ Informal testing

All parents of all children are automatically and 'informally' testing their children every day. It is only natural for parents to be comparing their child with others in their own family and with the children of relatives and friends. In fact, this informal 'testing' is the first test when considering detecting dyslexia in a child. The parents may be the first to notice there are differences – especially if something begins to show up before the child goes to school. Once at school it may be the other way around. The teacher may be the first to notice something and report to the parents that there is a possible problem.

The first and easiest step in this process of 'testing' is to record your natural everyday observations of your child's behaviour and interactions with you and other children and adults.

Signs to look out for

If your child is too young to go to school there are still signs you may be able to pick out that will alert you to the fact that he may have some difficulties at school. The symptoms and characteristics listed below are taken from an excellent list compiled for parents by the British Dyslexia Association.

Of course all children will show some of these signs some of the time. What is interesting for you to note is if any of these behaviours start to become consistent and persistent.

- speaking clearly later than expected
- jumbled phrases, eg 'cobbler's club' for 'toddler's club', 'teddy-dare' for 'teddy-bear'
- a quick 'thinker' and 'do-er'
- use of substitute words or 'near misses'
- mislabelling, eg lampshade for lamp post
- a lisp – 'duckth' for 'ducks'
- inability to remember the label for known objects, eg colours
- confused directional words, eg 'up/down' or 'in/out'
- excessive tripping, bumping into things and falling over nothing
- enhanced creativity – often good at drawing, good sense of colour
- obvious 'good' and 'bad' days for no apparent reason
- aptitude for constructional or technical toys, eg bricks, puzzles, Lego blocks, remote control for TV and video, computer keyboards
- enjoys being read to but shows no interest in letters or words
- difficulty learning nursery rhymes
- difficulty with rhyming words, eg 'cat mat fat'
- difficulty with odd-one-out, eg 'cat mat pig fat'
- did not crawl – was a 'bottom shuffler'
- difficulty with 'sequence', eg coloured bead sequence
- appears 'bright' – seems an enigma
- mixed laterality – no preference for left or right
- inability to follow a sequence of instructions
- does not pay attention
- cannot sit still
- disturbs others
- becomes irritable and shows frustration easily
- stubborn
- does not finish work

- immature
- acts out ideas rather than using words

■ Formal testing

The point of intervention

Normally the symptoms of an actual learning disability will not be measurable in terms of a test before a child is at school because, for the pre-school child, there are no standards against which to measure any lack of ability.

In addition, it is a fact that children develop at very different rates. Some walk before they can crawl while others are very delayed in getting mobile. The same may be true of speech – one child may be speaking in full sentences much too early and another will be far behind in making clear sounds and communicating with words.

Once in school children are expected to follow a normal course of development, within acceptable limits. If a child starts to fall behind this norm either his parents or teacher will suggest he be tested for a learning disability.

The term point of intervention is a way of saying that there is a point where the difference your child is showing from some accepted norm in a particular area is large enough to require further investigation. This point is not fixed. It varies from school to school and there are many different opinions about where it should be set.

All parents and many teachers know that the decision to have a young child tested is complex one and one that should not be taken casually. Testing often implies there is something wrong or something different. Some parents and teachers will wait as long as possible before having a child tested in the hope that he will catch up and reduce the difference he is showing in certain areas. Other parents and teachers are of the opinion that the sooner the child is tested the sooner he can begin receiving treatment and perhaps avoid more serious problems with learning later in his schooling.

This may be confusing for parents who seek advice from more than one source. They may receive conflicting recommendations about what is best for their child. By becoming aware of both points of view, parents can make their own judgement and arrive at the right decision about when to intervene and have a test done on their child or when to begin treatment.

Sometimes a teacher may say to parents who want their child to be tested, 'Well, let's just wait a while and see if your son gets through this phase and catches up.' Sometimes it will be the reverse with the school insisting and the parents feeling it is not the right time. At this point it is always a matter of weighing up the advantages and disadvantages of introducing your child to the world of tests and special classes.

Labelling a child dyslexic

Even among experts there is disagreement about whether a child should be tested and identified as dyslexic. Some argue that the label 'dyslexic' becomes a self-fulfilling term and that as soon as a child is diagnosed as such he ceases to try to overcome his learning disabilities and succumbs to being classified as learning disabled. Others argue the opposite and say that if a child who is dyslexic is not identified and taken out of the normal classroom situation and given special attention that child will become even more learning disabled. Failure to identify a potentially dyslexic child may mean he never has a chance to catch up and be re-integrated into the appropriate class level for his age.

What is testing based on?

Before we describe the tests it is good to take a slight side-step and look at the approach of the tests. All testing for dyslexia is based on the following general definition: 'Dyslexia is a certain set of symptoms (which vary from one definition to another) coming from one or a number of different causes.' This means that the results of any test for dyslexia will depend entirely on the test's definition of dyslexia.

What a test can (and cannot) do

A test only tests for what it is looking for. This may sound obvious (or strange), but it is a warning about what you can expect any test for dyslexia to tell you.

There are two main limitations in all testing done for dyslexia. Firstly, if a test is not testing for a particular symptom of dyslexia these symptoms will not show up in the test results, even if your child has them and you as a parent can see they are there. For example, a test for reading ability will not show up any symptoms of difficulties with maths. This gives rise to the anguish some parents feel when their child is tested and the results show that he is *not* dyslexic. In this situation the symptoms of dyslexia being used as a measure for dyslexia (and being tested for in that particular test) were not present in your child. Therefore, this particular test will conclude that your child is not dyslexic. Meanwhile you know all too well how much your child is struggling at school.

Secondly, a test for dyslexia is usually a test for a particular set of symptoms and much less often a test for a particular *cause* of those symptoms. This means that even if a test confirms that your child has symptoms of dyslexia, there is nothing in the test results to indicate how to address the cause of those symptoms. Very often another set of tests needs to be done to determine the possible cause of the symptoms.

When is dyslexia not dyslexia?

As mentioned above, the number or mixture of symptoms that are taken to suggest dyslexia is not standard but varies according to the test being used. Some tests will choose a certain level of symptoms. Others may choose another set or level of the same symptoms. Statistics are used to separate out those who are dyslexic. This is not particular to dyslexia testing.

The majority of tests for dyslexia will look for the symptoms of dyslexia that a child produces under certain controlled circumstances. On the basis of results from these tests an opinion will be given as to whether a child is dyslexic or not. The results show how well the child is able to take the test. However, dyslexic children are known to be afraid of tests and to perform less well under test conditions. This is another factor to take into account when test results seem to vary for the same child. If a child takes the same test on different days the results can vary significantly enough for him to be diagnosed dyslexic on one day on not on the other.

Despite the above limitations on the testing of dyslexia, your child may be officially diagnosed as dyslexic and tests will need to be done. Below is an overview of the various forms of formal testing that are available and what they can offer.

Differential diagnosis

Perhaps the commonest and most easily administered test is the 'differential diagnosis' test. This is normally administered by an educational psychologist who will do a series of tests to determine in which areas of school work your child is statistically significantly behind the 'norm', ie the areas that your child is finding more difficult than an average child of his age in his class.

Levels set for all areas for all ages are used as a standard. By comparing your child to these standards a 'profile' can be drawn of him. When this is compared with the profile of an average, normal child of the same age it is possible to see where your child's performance in the test differs from this expected norm.

The educational psychologist may test your child in the following areas:

- his academic performance (compared with that of the average child)
- his use of language
- his memory and attention span
- his visual-spatial abilities
- his motor skills (coordination) and 'fine-motor' skills (ability to make precise movements)

There are many different standard tests used for this form of psychological and educational testing. Some of the names you may hear mentioned in connection with these tests are the Aston Index, WISC III and LPAD (Learning Potential Assessment Device).

These tests may not tell you anything you did not already know. They may be useful to tell you just *how much* below normal your child is in a particular area. They may give the statistical 'proof' that your child is not performing normally in certain areas. Some people may go ahead and use the information from such a test to conclude that your child is dyslexic. Others may say that more tests need to be done before any such conclusion can be drawn.

Paediatric testing

The next logical test to be done after a differential diagnosis has shown that your child is under-achieving in some areas, is to determine whether a physical problem with hearing, vision or brain function could be causing his difficulties.

As well as testing for general health problems, a paediatrician will check your child's:

- nervous system and brain functions
- development and growth
- hearing
- vision
- sense of balance and motor functions

The testing will usually begin with testing of functions of the sense organs. Your child's performance in these tests will be compared with a set of 'normal' functions, in much the same way that your child's academic performance was compared with a set of norms.

If significant differences are found, this can be taken as an indication that there might be structural problems with the brain or sense organs. However, apart from the gross symptoms of malformation in the structure of the brain or sense organs, which are relatively easy to detect and record, it is quite difficult to test for structural problems directly in the nervous system and sense organs. This means that even though tests may show that there are differences between how your child's brain and sense organs function and how those of a 'normal' child of the same age function, the tests will not necessarily be able to show what is causing these differences.

If there is evidence from a paediatric test that your child has suffered some form of brain damage or if there is some other known structural cause of brain malfunction, then your child's dyslexic symptoms may be directly attributable to these causes.

Further testing

If there is no evidence or medical history of brain damage, no evidence of gross structural problems with the sense organs, and no significant difference from a normal child's performance in these tests, there are two further possibilities for what is causing your child's dyslexic symptoms.

The first possibility is that a structural problem which the present tests have not been able to detect may be causing the symptoms. The second is that it is not a *structural* problem at all but a *functional* problem with the brain and/or sense organs.

If you are faced with these two possibilities, a choice has to be made about how much further testing can or should be done on your child. The reasons for further testing are:

- to try and find the underlying structural cause of the symptoms
- to try and find out more precisely what the functional problems are so that appropriate treatments can be found to correct them

There are forms of dyslexia treatment available where testing for auditory and visual sensitivities is carried out and interpreted in a different way from the standard tests available from medical doctors or optometrists. These more detailed tests can reveal functional problems in the sense organs which can be treated with specific training for these organs. (For more information, *see* the sections on visual and auditory dysfunctions, pages 48–52.)

As each case of dyslexia is different, no common recommendation can be made and each child's needs must be assessed individually.

Psychological testing

Other tests are available that do not focus on the sense organs themselves but on the processing of the information received by the senses. These tests are based on the idea that there are other factors that can influence the functioning of a child's brain and sense organs.

It is well known that our psychological state at any moment can affect how we perceive the world and how we use our brains. So psychological testing is another avenue that can be explored for your dyslexic child. This is usually considered when the behaviour of a child is showing differences from a set of norms for behaviour.

If your child, in addition to his learning difficulties, is behaving in ways that seem beyond what might be considered normal or acceptable at home or in the classroom, a psychological test might be suggested in order to:

- check for any physical and postural imbalances that may be having an effect on your child's emotions, reactions, memory and ability to pay attention

- look into your child's psychological make up to see if there are any contributing factors. For example:
  - is he more afraid than the average child?
  - is he afraid of failing, with no trust in his own abilities?
  - does he have low self-esteem?
  - is he more withdrawn than would be considered normal?
  - is he rebellious and resisting control?
  - is he suffering from chronic depression?
  - is he subject to mood swings and disorders?
  - does he suffer from psychosomatic illnesses – headaches, stomach complaints, skin disorders, frequent colds?

The psychologist may also want to assess environmental factors that could be influencing your child's behaviour:

- his psychological environment at home, at school, and with his friends
- his physical environment in terms of chemical sensitivities or antigens which may be causing reactions or allergies that affect his behaviour and responsiveness

There is a great deal of variation in how comprehensive such psychological tests may be. Ideally any psychological test would include as many of the above-mentioned variables as possible, but this is not always the case.

Summary

1 There is no standard, objective, commonly-agreed-upon set of criteria for dyslexia presently available. In the end, the decision as to whether the differences from a norm shown in a test imply your child is dyslexic will be based upon the subjective judgement of the testing person or the persons who designed the test. Because the symptoms of dyslexia are so varied and mixed, there are no clear-cut boundaries which define where dyslexia begins. This can be exasperating when you need to make a decision about your child based on testing.

2 Any testing for dyslexia is usually an ordeal for your child, and may also be for you.

3 After an initial test for dyslexia, it is advisable to consider carefully which additional tests you want to put your child through. What is to be avoided is the situation where a child has a whole series of tests and treatments in the hope that one of them will prove positive or work. As mentioned at the beginning of this section, 'Taking stock' and 'Deciding what you want to achieve' are very important steps to take. It happens all too often that parents, in their enthusiasm and desire to help, will subject their child to so many tests that at a certain point, out of self-protection, the child will refuse any more help and retreat behind a wall of non-cooperation and withdrawal.

■ HELPING YOUR CHILD

Once your child has been diagnosed dyslexic, the next step is to look at what you can practically do. In the following sections you will find advice on how you can help both your child – at home, outside the home, and at school – and yourself. The suggestions offered are not meant to be a replacement for any treatment for dyslexia. They will often, however, make a big difference to how your child responds to any orthodox treatment he is given.

A selection of the treatments available for dyslexia is provided to help you assess which one would be most appropriate for your child.

■ In the home

- Be sensitive to your child's emotions and feelings and his reactions to having a disability – and talk about these with him, if at all possible. Find a way of talking to other people about your child's disability that you feel comfortable with so that he does not get the feeling that you have something to hide or are embarrassed about.

- Be aware of your own emotions when discovering your child has a learning disability. Try not to let these personal emotions influence your judgements about what your child needs. (*See* 'Helping Yourself', pages 31–41.)

- Encourage your child to develop skills and talents in areas where he is *not* disabled – sport, drama, artistic and creative pursuits, perhaps – where he may show talents that are not limited by not being able to read, spell or do maths.

- Arrange your child's physical environment to make it easier for him to study at home. Plan set times when he does his homework and keep his schedule as consistent as possible.

- Find a balance between support for your child in coping with his disability and over-protectiveness that can create dependency and need.

- Recognize and be aware that sometimes when a child who is disabled is undergoing treatment and learning to read or become more competent in a skill, he may be afraid that he will change and become someone else. If there has been a strong pattern of dependency before the treatment begins, he may become concerned that his parents will not love him any more once he is no longer so disabled.

- Recognize behaviours that are a 'smoke-screen' for a disability in your child. He may behave in exaggerated and provoking ways only in an attempt to distract you from making demands that require him to perform skills at which he feels he will fail.

- Be sensitive to the natural tendency to lower expectations in all areas when making demands on a learning disabled child. Obviously in areas where there are difficulties, expectations must be adjusted appropriately. But in other areas, where a child has no disabilities, be careful not to apply the same lower level of expectation. This will only weaken a child's already fragile feelings of self-worth.

- Practise patience with your dyslexic child. Being anxious, concerned or impatient will only add to his feeling of insecurity and make his dyslexic symptoms worse.

- Encourage a dyslexic child's natural curiosity. Curiosity will help maintain the motivation to learn that is worn away by the difficulties he experiences in working with symbols.
- Give a dyslexic child the chance to find out things for himself. Encourage self-responsibility and independence. In the learning situation at home let the child lead and determine the pace rather than take the passive role.
- Help your child to relax. This is one of the simplest and most important things you can do to help your child. Because he has difficulty doing things that other children find easy, he will always have to work much harder and for longer in order to keep up with the teacher writing on the blackboard or to do his homework. The frustration and effort this takes cause headaches and tension. Your child may come home at the end of a day at school completely exhausted. The frustration he has not been able to express while at school may suddenly come bursting out the moment he gets home.

The release procedure

A simple but very effective relaxation technique that can help you to help your child is the Release Procedure. It was developed by Ron Davis at his Reading Research Council especially for dyslexic children who tend to become tense and to concentrate too hard to try and get things done. This procedure can also be used by you when you find yourself getting uptight and concerned and unable to let things go. It is best performed in an environment where there are as few distractions as possible.

Get comfortable. As comfortable as you can.
Make a loose fist, not too tight, just let your fingers curl into your palm.
Now think the thought 'open hand', and make the fist tighter.

Think the thought 'open hand' again, and make the fist even tighter.

Once more think the thought 'open hand', and make the fist really tight, tight all the way up to your elbow.

Now, without thought, simply let your hand go, let your fingers find their natural place.

Feel the feeling that goes down your arm, through your hand, all the way out to the tips of your fingers. That is the feeling of release. When the word 'release' is used, that feeling is what is meant.

The feeling of release is the same feeling as a sigh. Let out a sigh. Breathe in, hold it for a second, now let the air rush out of your mouth, with the 'hunnn' sound coming from your throat and chest. A little sigh puts the feeling of release in your upper chest. A great big sigh can spread that feeling all the way out to the tips of your fingers and toes. Let out a great big sigh, get that feeling all through your body. Now let that feeling linger, let that feeling remain in your body.

Close your eyes. Feel your toes, find where your toes are and feel them from the inside.

Hold your feeling of your toes and feel your fingers. Find where your fingers are and feel them from the inside.

Now expand your feeling from your toes all the way to your ankles, and from your fingers all the way to your wrists.

Now continue to expand your feeling from your toes all the way to your knees and from your fingers all the way to your elbows.

Continue all the way to your hips and shoulders.

Now all through your body, all the way up to your neck.

Now all through your neck and head, including your ears, all the way to the skin on the top of your head.

Now let out a great big sigh and flood your entire body with the feeling of release, all the way out to the tips of your fingers and toes.

Let that feeling of release remain in your body and, when it is comfortable to do so, allow your eyes to open.

Once your child has been able to experience clearly the feeling of release through his whole body then you can use a shorthand form of this procedure whenever he gets tense or has a headache. Just ask him to let out a big sigh, really big and deep from the bottom of his stomach. This will have the effect of pouring the feeling of release right through his body. It sounds very simple but it is remarkably effective.

■ At school

As far as possible establish good relationships with your child's school and teachers. There are two possible scenarios:

1 The school and teachers are supportive and cooperative and want to find ways for your child to adapt and work with his disabilities.
2 The school and/or teachers are not sympathetic for whatever reason and are not willing or able to provide support and encouragement for your child.

Scenario 1

In this fortunate situation you can help to maintain this positive approach by staying in close contact with the teachers. This may be in the form of:

- regular meetings to discuss your child's progress at school
- meetings at school with teachers and parents of other learning disabled children to support each other and cooperate in coordinating services for the children
- keeping your child's teacher updated on how you are supporting your child at home
- reporting on such things as:
  - your child's successes outside of school
  - changes in your child's attitude and behaviour that may be important for the teacher to take into account when teaching him in class
  - changes in family circumstances and any other influences that may be affecting your child's difficulties at school
  - new information you may have researched about learning disabilities and their treatment

Of course all of this contact with your child's teachers and school should be done in complete openness. Your child should never be left with the feeling that you are somehow in collaboration with the school 'behind his back'.

Scenario 2

In the situation where you find little support and cooperation for your child's disabilities there are two options to consider:

- moving your child to another school where more support and cooperation is available
- finding ways to change the attitude of the school and teachers

If you decide on the second option there are several things you can do:

- Find out about your legal rights and insist they be met.
- Get together with other parents and work towards changing the attitude of the school and teachers (do remember, though, to always try and put yourself in the position of the school and teachers before making any negative judgements – they may be operating under certain limitations and restrictions).
- Try to find possible reasons why the school is not cooperative; for example:
  - it may be unable, rather than unwilling to cooperate with you because of shortage of resources;
  - teachers may not be fully aware of all the options in helping learning disabled children.
- Make the first gesture by offering to help at the school and build up relationships in this way before making demands for your child.

Any action you can take to influence your child's school or teachers will cost you extra time and energy. It is important in all these sorts of decisions to be clear on your priorities. Bear in mind that it is unwise to communicate negative judgements directly to a teacher or school. Whatever you may be feeling it does not help to blame the school. They will be doing whatever they can to the best of their ability within the limitations they have to work with. It does not help you or them to be critical and angry about their lack of cooperation in helping your child.

Every parent has only so much energy and time available – establishing the right balance between pushing for what your child needs at school and accepting the inherent limitations in a situation is always an artful matter. This will be discussed further in 'Helping Yourself'.

■ Outside home and school

The general guidelines to follow in this area are:

- Find activities outside home and school which your child enjoys and where he can establish, maintain and build his self-esteem, self-confidence and identity as a person who is not disabled.
- Cultivate activities that challenge and develop your child's natural talents.
- Look for activities and social circles that will not be threatening to your child and which do not require him to perform in areas where he feels unsure about himself.
- Be aware of how your child changes as he grows. Changes in emotions, needs and interests can happen very quickly. At certain ages in the development of a dyslexic child there are often turning or crisis points when everything can change very suddenly. (For a more detailed description of these changes, *see* pages 95–106.) Try to be aware of these moments and adapt yourself and your child's life as much as possible to accommodate these changes.
- Do not insist that your child continues to do something he has enjoyed in the past when it is clear that he is going through a process of change. On the other hand, consistency

and structure and predictability are very much needed by dyslexic children. Consider carefully any changes that you do make in your child's activities and schedule and discuss them as much as possible in advance with him.

As you can see there are no hard and fast rules that can be applied to helping your child to live with and adapt to his learning disabilities. It is always a matter of remaining sensitive and in communication and maintaining as much balance and humour as possible throughout the difficult process of coming to terms with a disability.

■ HELPING YOURSELF

The idea that helping yourself could be part of helping your dyslexic child may seem strange at first. You may have become so used to having all your attention and energy focused on helping your child adapt to his difficulties that you have got into the habit of hardly noticing what you yourself are thinking or feeling. The thought of considering yourself or accommodating your own needs may never have crossed your mind. If so, now is the time to take a moment to do just that. Although this is said lightly, there is a serious side to the idea of helping yourself as part of helping your disabled child. There are two realities you must take into account:

- You will not be able to truly help your child in his disability if you are not at ease and at peace with yourself.
- What you have been doing up until now to help your child may be the very thing that is preventing you from being at peace with yourself and your child's disability.

A vicious circle can develop in the relationship between a dyslexic child and his parents that makes it impossible for him to be helped. The simplest version of this double bind is that a dyslexic child's disabilities become the context or structure of the relationship between parents and child. How you are with your child and what you talk about and share forms the basis of working on the disability. Anything that might correct the disability will then be felt as unfamiliar and therefore a possible threat to the dynamic of the relationship. This could affect the chances of a dyslexic child being relieved of his disability.

There are many degrees and variations of this connection between parents and a dyslexic child. It is inevitable to some degree. No one needs to feel guilty that such a dynamics exists. But is important to be aware of this often unconscious element in the relationship. With this awareness, steps can be taken to break the vicious circle that can keep a dyslexic child trapped in his disability for his whole life.

▓ 1 Establishing a Point of Reference

Whether or not you are aware of the dynamics within your relationship with your child, the first step in helping yourself is to establish a Point of Reference for yourself in relation to your child's dyslexia. To be useful, a Point of Reference must be:

- independent of how you are feeling or thinking at any particular moment
- fixed and constant (something that you can use to measure other ideas against)
- visible and easily accessible at any moment

Almost any idea, belief or principle can be taken and used as a Point of Reference, which can be likened to a direction. Take the compass point North, for example – it is always there and if you are travelling northwards it will help you make decisions about which way to go. A Point of Reference is a way of orienting yourself in relation to everything you have to do. If it can be maintained, it allows a certain integrity and consistency to come into your life.

Ideals and good causes, beliefs in a higher principle, a burning passion or hobby, a particular point of view – these are just a few examples of what can be taken on as a Point of Reference. If it is to be effective however it must also be present and available in your life. Some vague notion of wanting to live a good and true life will not be sufficient to help you in making decisions and organizing priorities. The benefit and satisfactions of maintaining a Point of Reference must be felt for it to be useful. The meaning of your life will be directly influenced by the Point of Reference you have chosen.

In families where a dyslexic child is having difficulties it is quite common that the problem of dealing with the dyslexia becomes the Point of Reference for the parents and therefore for the whole family. Rather than being a part of a larger meaning that gives direction, the dyslexia and its problems become the guiding principle around which everything revolves and in the light of which decisions are taken and choices made.

We all need and choose Points of Reference, whether we are aware of it or not. This is simply because without such reference and direction we would be lost in a sea of possibilities and not know what to choose. So once we have found a Point of Reference, all choices made will tend to be those that preserve the meaning or way of seeing things that our Point of Reference provides. When parents choose a child's learning difficulties as the Point of Reference for themselves and their families, even for the very best of reasons, it will inevitably involve them in making choices that could maintain that Point of Reference – and thus the very problem they are trying to solve – intact.

To summarize, it is important to:

- Be aware of adopting the demands of living with a dyslexic child as your Point of Reference since this may perpetuate the problem rather than solve it.
- Choose your Point of Reference *outside* the context of your child's dyslexia.
- Actively maintain and re-enact your Point of Reference as part of your daily life. Make sure you experience benefits and satisfactions from having made that particular choice.

Active re-affirmation of a Point of Reference other than your child's learning difficulties will bring the balance and distance you need as a parent. By directing some of your attention away from your child's needs you will be more effective in helping him find his own way of adapting to his difficulties. Without that distance you can 'fall into' the problem and your child will become dependent on you and never learn his own way in life.

Your Point of Reference needs to be more than just an idea or a goal, and to be effective it needs to be expressed in concrete actions and positive choices. Whatever system you have of allocating priorities to the various ways you use your time, it must include actions directly connected to maintaining your Point of Reference. By consciously allocating part of your time and energy to responding to this Point of Reference, the other areas of your life, including helping your child with his dyslexia, will fall into perspective.

■ 2 Understanding your responsibilities

If you are not aware of having a choice in managing the demands on your time and attention, this should be the first priority for you to establish in helping your child with his dyslexia. Without the ability to make choices in a particular area of your life, you will not be able to exercise any responsibility in that area.

Responsibility, in its simplest meaning, is not about being serious and concerned for something or someone. It is just the willingness and ability to control something. Controlling something only means being able to make something change or stop it from changing. This simple concept of what responsibility is and is not can have a very powerful effect when it comes to helping your child cope with learning difficulties caused by dyslexia.

Parents who are not able to make choices about how to allocate their time and resources are not in a position to be responsible for helping their dyslexic child. And there are some parents who are so constrained. The problems arise when a parent in such a situation begins to feel responsible for his or her child without being in any way able to exercise that responsibility. That is a desperate situation to be in. By understanding the idea of what responsibility requires you can simply see which areas you can and cannot be responsible for. This can keep you from trying to attempt the impossible and feeling that you are somehow always failing.

3 Taking an emotional inventory

Fixed emotions or emotional reactions sometimes can become the Point of Reference we choose to live by. Becoming aware of our emotions always helps us to be more aware of what Points of Reference we have chosen and whether that Point of Reference is actually supporting the people in our lives that we care about.

Making an inventory or doing a 'stock take' of your present and past emotions can help you become aware of any particular emotion that may be acting as a Point of Reference for you. This is not always an easy task. It requires facing up to and acknowledging what you are feeling. You may consider that some of these feelings are not acceptable for parents – you in particular – to have.

To make this emotional inventory you have to ask for help from someone you trust and who you feel will not judge you for expressing your feelings. Your partner may not necessarily be the right person to choose. Many parents have found a chance to acknowledge their emotions in the context of a support group of other parents of dyslexic children. If this is not available and you feel you cannot do it by yourself then choose a person or group that will allow this opening of yourself to occur without any threat.

Checklist of emotions

To help you make your emotional inventory I have listed below a number of emotions that parents experience when confronted with the fact that their child is learning disabled. The first five are the ones most commonly felt and are listed in the order they usually occur.

Denial. You do not believe the test results of reports from school.
Anger. You do not want to accept that your child is the one to have dyslexia. Why him? Why you?
Depression. You have a child who will never be normal.
Acceptance resignation. You must get on with dealing with the new situation, find help, become active.
Hope. You begin to feel that maybe there is a way to help your child learn.

Parents may stop at any one of these stages or may fluctuate between different emotions depending on how their child is adapting to his learning disability. Other emotions that may arise later or simultaneously are.

Guilt. You feel that as a parent you are somehow to blame for your child's difficulties. For mothers this may involve concern that she may have done something during her pregnancy to damage the child. It may involve not feeling adequate as a parent to bring up such a demanding child.
Embarrassment/shame/awkwardness. You do not know what to tell your family or friends about your child's disability. The same emotion may also be directed towards your child.
Anger or rage. This may be directed at yourself or at 'them' – school, psychologists, parents of children who are not learning disabled. It may even be directed at your dyslexic child.
Frustration. This may be caused by many different things: you may not be able to get a clear message about your child's learning difficulties from school or 'experts'; you may not be able to get the help and recognition that your child needs; or you feel

unable to help your child however hard you try and he cannot seem to cooperate with your need to help.

Despair. This occurs when the frustration becomes overwhelming and you cannot see a way forward.

Grief. You mourn for the child you had been longing for and who has somehow disappeared.

Pity. This can be either for yourself or for your child, or for both.

Resentment. This can be towards your child, yourself, doctors, teachers and even towards other children who are not disabled, both your own and others.

Betrayal. Whatever hopes you had for your child and yourself and your family have been destroyed or denied and you feel justified in blaming others or your particular situation for the feelings that come with unfulfilled expectations.

Feelings of being exploited, abused emotionally and/or physically. This again is related to your expectation of how you *should* be feeling, which is not validated or supported by your experience.

Fear. This can manifest as a vague fear of the future and what will happen to your child; fear of failing to look after your child; fear of your child who is rebelling and out of control; fear for your child who is so frustrated he may do something to hurt himself or others; fear of losing contact with a child who is withdrawing.

Disgust. This can be with yourself for failing to produce a normal child or for giving up trying to help him, or with your child who is challenging all your cherished principles and beliefs.

Sadness. Sometimes this can just come over you without any particular apparent outside cause. These emotions are often very deep and may not be directly linked with your child and his difficulties, but he somehow triggers off these feelings in you that you can do nothing about.

Loneliness. You feel there is no one to turn to who can understand your child or your own situation as a parent of a learning disabled child.

Helplessness. You have tried everything for so long and nothing is working.

Panic. You do not know what to do and become unable to make decisions or see clearly.

Hurt. Feelings can be easily hurt when the love and caring we offer is denied, ignored and rejected. An almost inevitable part of living with others is that we get hurt and feel emotional pain. Trying to avoid getting hurt does not help and can make communications with your child and other members of the family even more difficult. Finding a way to live with being hurt and to remain loving without withdrawing is the challenge.

Although I have listed all the negative emotions first, positive emotions are experienced too. It is very important to acknowledge and affirm these and to find others who share these emotions and allow you to express them.

Deep love and acceptance. It is sometimes harder to express these two emotions than all the others, especially when you are feeling hurt and depressed by what has happened.

Pride and enjoyment. You see your child overcoming his difficulties or accepting his limitations without being sorry for himself. You can celebrate his achievements with him. You accept that the dyslexia is just something that has to be dealt with rather than a major problem.

Make use of the above checklist by:

- identifying which emotions apply to you
- trying to express more exactly how you experience these emotions with someone you trust
- noticing how these emotions affect your life, the others in your family and your attitudes

■ **Further steps**

If you feel able to take the above three steps you may also want to go further and express how you feel about the disability itself.

This involves a much more specific description and you may not feel able or ready to do this at this moment. When dealing with feelings about your child's disability it is helpful to understand the following important distinction: what you feel about your child's *disabilities* is not the same as what you feel about *your child*. Once you make this distinction it often releases the emotions that you have held back because you thought it was unacceptable to feel certain things about your disabled child.

There is one further emotional area which needs to be acknowledged and accepted. These emotions are in some ways even more difficult to bring out and look at because they are not directly connected with the child but relate specifically to the parents. If you yourself had difficulties at school and some form of learning disability, all the emotions attached to this from the past may be re-activated by seeing your child go through similar experiences. You may have gone to great lengths to suppress painful childhood memories and may not be willing to have these old wounds re-opened. A conflict can be generated when you are torn between having to care for a learning disabled child and needing to forget your own past traumas related to learning. It could reach a point when you want to deny your child's difficulties simply because they are too much a reminder of your own childhood suffering.

I do not mean to imply that you cannot help your child unless all your emotions are laid out and fully expressed. It is certainly not the case that you have to make this emotional inventory before you can help your child with his difficulties. But I do feel that it is beneficial to be aware of the emotions connected with your child's disability – or with a disability you may have or have had yourself – otherwise these emotions may interfere with the help you are able to give.

The final point to make here is that dyslexic children are extremely sensitive to the emotions and feelings of other people. They will often be able to tell you what you are feeling before you are aware of it yourself!

It is interesting to consider for a moment why dyslexics can 'read' people so well. Their ability to think in pictures and their heightened awareness of what is going on around them in the environment will be discussed later in the book, but the combination of these two talents creates an uncanny ability to know what someone else is feeling.

When someone thinks in pictures, very little internal conversation is going on in that person's head. This means he is not so distracted by mental analysis and judgements or by the words a person is saying. Instead he sees the person as a whole, in a picture. The picture he sees is often different from the words that the other person is saying – as a dyslexic he tends to find it easier to read non-verbal communication and relies on this far more than someone who finds words easy to manage. He is also very aware of those signals and messages from the environment that are not filtered through words. Picture thinking also happens extremely fast, much faster than words. So a dyslexic will know what you are going to say before you have said it and tell you what you are feeling before you have had time to formulate the words.

This being the case, it is all the more important that you are clear about what you are feeling and that what you communicate to your child is clear and as congruent as possible with your emotions. It is far better to tell your child what you are feeling than to try and hide your feelings behind a more superficial message.

Dyslexic children are disturbed by confusion. As you will read later in this book, confusion is one of the main contributing factors to the symptoms of dyslexia. Simply put, the symptoms of dyslexia are one of the results of a dyslexic child's unsuccessful attempt to overcome confusion in his environment. Conflicting messages and signs from someone as important as a parent will lead a child to be uncertain about what is going on in his emotional environment. This will cause a reaction in a dyslexic child that can make the dyslexic symptoms worse.

Making a plan of action

Any situation where a child has a disability and is no longer a 'normal' child brings with it its own set of demands and adjustments. Emotions can sometimes get in the way of good judgement. The needs of the child may become obscured by powerful feelings from the parents. It can happen that parents want to do something for their child more as a reaction to what *they* are feeling than as part of helping their child with his learning disability.

Because emotions play such an important role in helping your dyslexic child, there is a real need for a concrete plan that is realistic. Objective support from someone not directly involved in your family situation is always most welcome at these moments. Your plan of action should include the following elements:

- help you can give your child
- help you can give yourself
- help you can ask for from people specializing in dyslexia treatment

The following section on orthodox treatments for dyslexia is in no way meant to be comprehensive, but covers examples of different forms of treatment chosen from the many possibilities. This choice is meant to give you an idea of how to assess any particular treatment that you may encounter in your search to help your child.

TREATMENT

Choosing a treatment

Before deciding on a treatment for your child, consider the following factors:

- What are the goals of this particular treatment? Is there a fixed time period in which the treatment will be given or is it open-ended?

- What will treatment cost? The costs in both money and time need to be considered. If a course of treatment puts too much financial strain on a family, an extra, often unconscious, burden of expectation is placed on the dyslexic child. The child will feel he must progress and improve in order to justify the expense. If a treatment cannot be given freely to a child, with no conditions attached, it may be better not to start the treatment at all. That is not to say that goals cannot be agreed upon between child and parent, but very often, parents' hidden expectations can sabotage any hope of a treatment helping the child because of the pressure he feels to succeed.

- What will be the prognosis if treatment is not given? It is always good to weigh up the advantages and disadvantages of starting a treatment. Try not to be forced into taking action by feeling obliged to comply with someone else's expectations and demands. This is especially true when demands are made on parents to give medication to their child for dyslexia.

- What is the availability of trained therapists or remedial teachers to deliver the treatment, and is the child's school cooperative about giving him time off to attend treatments? Some treatments also require follow-up support and input from teachers or parents. Is the school willing to do this? If this suppport is not possible to arrange or maintain, consider the implications of this very carefully before beginning a treatment.

- How effective has the treatment been for others?

■ Before starting treatment

Find out as much as possible about the expected results of any treatment – what criteria are used to assess the results and what time commitment is required to achieve them? And make sure you know of any other conditions that need to be fulfilled. This research is particularly useful because of the many new ideas that continue to appear about the treatment of dyslexia.

If at all possible find out the credentials of anyone offering a new therapy or treatment. Visit the therapist to discuss your child's needs before making any long-term commitment of time and money.

It is a good idea to ask for a list of references from clients who have already been treated by this method. If you can contact these people and talk to them you will get an indication of what results to expect and what demands this particular form of treatment will make on your child. If a therapist is not able to supply you with a list of references be cautious before spending any time and money on that particular therapist's services.

■ Rating a treatment

Two standards are used whenever a treatment needs to be rated. One is the 'Removal of Symptoms', the other is the 'Removal of Cause(s)'. A treatment that is very effective at removing symptoms may, in fact, be ineffective at removing the cause of the symptoms.

So when rating any treatment of dyslexia the first question to ask is, 'Which sort of treatment is this? Is it a symptom-removal treatment or a cause-removal treatment?' Obviously it is always better to remove a cause than to remove only the symptoms, leaving the cause in place. Any treatment working with the cause of dyslexia would therefore have a higher rating than a treatment that works only with symptoms.

Within cause-removal treatments a further scale or gradient can be used to arrive at a rating. It divides treatments into those that deal with one single cause and those that include many possible causes. These opposite approaches roughly correspond to the two different understandings of how things work in our lives.

One picture suggests that our lives are made up of an intricate weave of intertwined patterns of cause and effect, with many levels of complexity. This is often associated with what might be called the 'eastern' or 'oriental' or holistic point of view. The other picture proposes that all that happens to us can be explained in terms of a mechanical affair involving separate, unrelated entities that exist in discrete independence but occasionally interact with one other. This has been labelled the 'western' or scientific, reductionistic, materialistic point of view.

Some treatments for the cause of dyslexia are very specific and directed to one particular function or organ in a child's body. Other treatments try to take into account a wide range of variables that could be contributing to a child's symptoms. It is known that there is a wide variation in symptoms between one dyslexic child and another. This suggests that a number of different causes may be operating in any moment to create a set of symptoms.

Any treatment that is able to account for a wide range of possible causes is more likely to be effective than a treatment that focuses on only one. A holistic treatment that takes the whole of the child's life into account would therefore receive a higher rating.

▓ Compatibility of different treatments

Many parents have questions about whether it is possible for their child to undergo a variety of different treatments for dyslexia at the same time. They want to know if one course of treatment will interfere with the results produced by another form of treatment. The following general guidelines apply.

1 If your child is undergoing treatment for his *symptoms* of dyslexia he will probably be given a specific Individualized Education Programme (IEP). (For a full explanation of IEP *see* pages 45–7.) These training programmes usually depend heavily on a set of training patterns and techniques. If a child changes from one IEP to another with a different set of training patterns, he may become confused by the new and conflicting instructions.

2 Any treatment which aims to correct a specific *cause* of dyslexic symptoms could have a beneficial effect on any training programme for removing dyslexic *symptoms*. This is because most treatments that work with specific causes of dyslexia try to remove obstructions in the child's ability to receive, process and repeat information – written or verbal. As these obstructions are removed, a training programme for removing symptoms would be helped by this improvement in functioning.

3 Whenever a child undergoes treatment for the cause of dyslexia, there should always be a period of time allowed after the treatment for its effects to take hold and bear fruit and for the child's body and senses to readjust and readapt. If another form of treatment is begun too soon or coincident with the first treatment, the beneficial effects of both treatments could be affected.

4 If a child is required to adapt and adjust too quickly, or if too many forces of change are working at any one moment, there is a danger that the child will simply resist all the treatments. This is his way of protecting himself from the overwhelming demands.

Symptom-removal treatments

In general, a treatment for the symptoms of dyslexia involves the following steps:

- making an assessment of the symptoms present
- designing a training programme to help a child adapt to, compensate for and/or overcome the specific difficulties he is having in the various processes involved in managing language and symbols – either written or spoken
- carrying out re-assessments at various times during the treatment to measure the reduction in symptoms

Individualized Education Programmes (IEPs)

A general term for this form of training programme is 'Individualized Education Programme'. IEPs are most often found in special education programmes offered by schools, colleges and private tutors. After assessing a child's strengths and weaknesses, the special education teacher will design an IEP outlining the specific skills the child needs to develop as well as appropriate learning activities that will build on his strengths. Many effective learning activities engage several skills and senses. For example, in learning to spell and recognize words, a student may be asked to see, say, write, and spell each new word.

Special education teachers also identify the types of tasks the child is able to perform and the senses that function well. By using the senses that are intact and bypassing the disabilities, many children can develop needed skills. These 'specific remediation techniques', as they are sometimes called, are so common and varied there is no way to describe them all in any detail.

The Orton-Gillingham approach   One name that is often associated with such training programmes is the Orton-Gillingham Academy. They describe their approach as a language-based, multi-sensory, structured, sequential, cumulative, cognitive and flexible programme. Because it is more a philosophy about the treatment of dyslexia than a system, it has been adapted into many different forms.

To give an idea of how an IEP treats the symptoms of dyslexia, two examples are given below.

Reading Recovery Programme   This is an example of a simple, straightforward remedial programme to help children who are backward in reading. It involves the following steps:

- re-reading two or more familiar books
- independent reading of the previous day's book, of which the teacher takes a running record or miscue analysis
- letter identification if necessary
- writing a story that the child has composed
- reassembling a story using pieces of text that have been cut up and pasted on to pieces of card

- introducing a new story to the child
- reading a new book

Speech therapy Therapy for speech and language disorders focuses on providing a stimulating but structured environment for hearing and practising language patterns. For example, the therapist may help a child with an articulation disorder to produce specific speech sounds. During an engaging activity, the therapist may talk about the toys, then encourage the child to use the same sounds or words. In addition, the child may watch the therapist make the sound, feel the vibration in the therapist's throat, then practise making the sounds before a mirror.

In some language disorders, the brain seems abnormally slow to process verbal information. Scientists are testing whether computers that talk can help teach children to process spoken sounds more quickly. The computer starts slowly, pronouncing one sound at a time. As the child gets better at recognizing the sounds and hearing them as words, the sounds are gradually speeded up to a normal rate of speech.

The results of using these remediation techniques are as varied as the techniques themselves. What is often a significant factor in the success of any of these programmes is the teacher or tutor offering the programme. The relationship between teacher and student often has more effect on a child's progress than which particular technique or approach is being used.

These treatments are designed to reduce dyslexic symptoms by producing other symptoms. The underlying cause of the symptoms is not necessarily addressed. Training, repetition and using the child's skills in other areas are the main hallmarks of this form of dyslexia treatment.

One other form of symptom-removal treatment – using drugs or medications – will be considered as part of a later section (*see* pages 61–2).

■ **Cause-removal treatments**

The treatments described in this section are those which attempt to deal with the cause of dyslexic symptoms. Usually one specific cause is selected and the treatment designed around this one cause. The treatments here have been roughly grouped according to which function has been selected as the cause of dyslexic symptoms.

Functional causes

Treatments for visual dysfunctions

Behavioural optometry   This is a special form of optometry that measures the capacity of the eyes to see and function properly. It involves more comprehensive tests on a child's eyes than normal optometry, often making use of kinesiology muscle testing as part of the assessment. Behavioural optometry allows specific imbalances in the muscles of the eye to be detected. Dyslexic children have significantly more trouble with this condition, often called 'Visual Directional Stress'. The child has difficulty turning his eyes and will move his head or whole body to compensate. This has a negative effect on reading and writing abilities.

Visual perceptual training   This form of vision therapy to correct eye muscle imbalances is based on the idea that visual skills are learned and therefore trainable. Exercises are given to the child to improve the use of his eye muscles and perceptual skills. In this way the child learns to use his visual system in a more efficient manner. This, in turn, facilitates learning as it helps him to receive, process and understand information more easily.

Irlen lenses   This therapy consists of supplying a learning disabled child with a set of glasses with coloured tinted lenses, specially selected for his particular needs. It is based on the scoptic sensitivity syndrome theories of Helen Irlen. Her theories state that sensitivity to full-spectrum light involves a structural brain deficit so that signals sent to the brain are inappropriately processed, resulting in perceptual problems. Therefore, light with all colours present (full-spectrum light) would distort what is perceived and processed by the brain.

Spectral modification, using Irlen coloured filters, minimizes or eliminates certain colours from full-spectrum light. Research has shown that individuals with Irlen filters can improve reading speed, fluency, comfort, comprehension and attention span while at the same time reducing strain, fatigue and the need for frequent breaks.

Lightwave stimulation This neuro-sensory development programme improves an individual's ability to absorb light energy so that the brain can function more efficiently. It is also used to treat scoptic sensitivity syndrome (see above). A standard treatment involves short daily sessions for 20 days. A child is first assessed to determine his visual field of awareness (how much light he can absorb from the natural environment). The treatment itself involves sitting in a darkened room listening to music and watching wavebands of light in colours that are likely to be beneficial for that child.

Children undergoing this treatment have found improvements in their learning and organizing abilities as well as a reduction in the stress and tension that can make other dyslexic symptoms worse.

Visualizing and Verbalizing for Language Comprehension and Thinking Programme – the Lindamood-Bell method This programme is for the treatment of a condition called Concept Imagery Disorder. Children with this disorder are weak in reading comprehension and oral language and have difficulty in following oral directions, problem solving, and processing both oral and written language. A child's ability to understand what he is reading is directly affected by imagery – or a lack of imagery. This programme aims to develop imagery, starting with one word and building up sentence by sentence to whole paragraphs and pages of text. The child then uses these images to create a whole picture from language which in turn develops his interpreting skills. He is helped to put these images into words using 'structure words' such as size, colour, number, meaning and background. This particular form of remedial counselling is carried out on a one-to-one basis.

Treatments for auditory dysfunctions

Auditory Discrimination in Depth (ADD) – the Lindamood-Bell method   The ADD (not to be confused with Attention Deficit Disorder) programme is based on the idea that underlying reading disorders come from an 'incompletely developed auditory conceptual function'. This auditory function or ability to compare and sequence sounds within spoken words is also called 'phoneme segmentation' or 'phonological awareness'.

According to this programme if you do not have a natural ability to process sounds in words you need to develop awareness of the phonemic structure in a direct and systematic manner. The programme starts by integrating the three senses of hearing, seeing and feeling into exploring sounds – how they are made, how they compare with each other and how they can be categorized. Students can use these three senses to perceive the identities, number and order of sounds within syllables, and thus learn accurate phonetic decoding and encoding skills.

The programme can also be used to prevent reading disabilities in primary school children. It has been found that auditory conceptual stimulation as a prelude to the reading/spelling process accelerates the development of these subjects and prevents disabilities.

Auditory Integration Training (AIT)   The underlying problem for many children with learning disabilities, attention deficit disorders and hyperactivity is often the impairment of auditory processing. Because their brains interpret, store and recall information differently or more slowly than others, they have problems understanding the world around them. Auditory Integration Training has been shown to help the underlying problem of processing sounds. By listening to music (processed through a special device called the Audiokinetron) through headphones the auditory system can be, in effect, reprogrammed. The Audiokinetron modulates the music by randomly varying the frequencies (low and high), the duration of sounds (long and short) and the volume (loud and soft) within comfort level limits. The training involves two 30-minute sessions a day for 10 days.

Tomatis method/Sound therapy The Tomatis theory states that the balance between the two hemispheres of the brain is of fundamental importance in overcoming dyslexia. Both hemispheres play a role in processing language, but the roles they play are different. The eye must combine with the power and the quality of the ear to make sense of the written sounds. This coordination happens easily when the left hemisphere deals primarily with audition and the right hemisphere deals primarily with vision. In dyslexia, the route which allows for analysis of sounds has been damaged. Sound therapy restores the functioning of this route and eliminates the cause of the problem. It does this by stimulating and exercising the ear, teaching it to receive and interpret sound in an efficient manner. Music is a highly organized series of sounds that the ear has to analyse. Therefore, listening to music is a excellent way for a child to learn how to perceive sounds in an organized fashion, or, in other words, to listen. The higher volume of sound to the right ear which is built into all sound therapy recordings means that the right ear is educated to be the directing ear. When this right ear dominance is achieved the problem of reversal will disappear.

The above treatments are focused on specific functions of the brain and sense organs concerned with the reception and processing of information. They involve retraining these functions to reduce the symptoms of dyslexia. The underlying cause of the dysfunction is not addressed in these treatments, but is assumed to be some 'malfunction' or delayed or interrupted development in a particular sense organ or function of the brain. Thus the fundamental cause of the dysfunction cannot be removed by these treatments.

One further treatment for an auditory dysfunction involves giving medication.

Levinson therapy   According to the theories of Dr Levinson, dyslexia is due to inner-ear dysfunction. It is known that anti-motion sickness medications help strengthen the inner ear's capacity to handle motion input and balance coordination output. Dr Levinson reasoned that these drugs can also improve the ability of the inner ear system to fine tune and process the total sensory input.

These medications do have the effect of reducing a wide range of dyslexic symptoms. Although they tend to work very well initially, their therapeutic effect eventually declines – and will also wear off if use of the medications is interrupted. By changing to another form of medication a favourable response can be started again.

The medications prescribed for this form of treatment for dyslexia include anti-motion sickness medications, antihistamines, stimulants, anti-depressants and vitamins.

This treatment identifies one of the sense organs as the cause of dyslexic symptoms. It does not address the underlying reason why the inner ear in dyslexics behaves in the way it does. In fact, the medications used to influence the inner ear's behaviour in this treatment do not allow the real cause of the inner ear's dysfunction to be corrected.

Physical causes

Treatments for specific body structures or organs The following manipulation therapies have been shown to have a beneficial effect on some dyslexic symptoms. The general thinking here is that if a child is out of balance in certain areas of his body it will have a negative influence on his energy and his ability to pay attention and function like a normal child.

Chiropractic Like all organs in the body, our brain has a nerve supply that controls and coordinates its activities. The portion of this nerve supply that emanates from the upper part of the neck can be disrupted when the bones of the spinal column get out of alignment (vertebral subluxation). Birth trauma; injuries sustained while learning to sit, crawl, stand or walk; childhood accidents and many other types of subtle damage to the delicate supportive tissues of the spine increase the likelihood of a vertebral subluxation. By minimizing vertebral subluxations, a child's body and mind can achieve their maximum potential. Chiropractic adjustments remove nerve pressure, increasing the flow of 'life energy' and enabling both the body and the mind to work at peak performance levels. The child may experience an increased attention span, an improved ability to focus, or a gentler, less restless nature.

Cranial osteopathy Poor functioning of the cranial mechanism can result in a structural imbalance in children, especially very young ones. This delicate mechanism involves the subtle movement of the cranial bones in response to the rhythm of the brain, which causes the 22 bones of the skull to move. This movement is reflected throughout the body in the form of a very subtle pulse – 10 to 12 times per minute. The muscles and the thin film covering all muscle and tissues are thus influenced by the structure of the body, and the body in turn influenced by the head.

Children with attention and learning difficulties are often

found to have limited movement in their cranial bones due to difficulties at birth. A child with this condition may have a poor appetite, suffer from colic, be unable to focus well, cry too much or need constant stimulation. As the child matures, learning disabilities may begin to appear. A very delicate form of osteopathy called cranial manipulation can be used to treat this problem. It can be performed at any age and results, especially in children, are usually rapid. The occipital bone of the skull is gently guided away from the atlas bone of the neck in order to restore motion. The movement is almost unnoticeable and is not painful.

Alexander technique   This is a technique for balancing and aligning the muscle systems in the body, particularly the spine and neck. It has beneficial effects on breathing and the sensory organs, improves the child's ability to pay attention or relax, and balances the energy levels in his body.

Neuro-developmental Delay Remediation (NDD)   In this treatment a sensory integration programme (reflex inhibition) is used to identify and correct motor and perceptual problems. It is sometimes referred to as the 'reflex inhibition programme'. It takes the client systematically through all the developmental stages involved in growing up – from a baby to an adult.

There are certain reflexes we all have when we are born – the so-called 'primitive reflexes'. These are necessary in the early stages of our development but when they are no longer needed they automatically become inhibited. These primitive reflexes are then replaced by the natural 'postural reflexes' that we all possess. But if the primitive reflexes are not inhibited and persist, this can produce symptoms of dyspraxia, dyslexia and ADD, bedwetting and thumb-sucking. These symptoms can be alleviated by a course of exercises practised at home.

Treatment is in the form of an initial assessment followed by a recommended Home Programme of Reflex Inhibition movements to inhibit the inappropriate primitive reflexes.

The above treatments, by adjusting the child's body and training its reflexes to be optimum and fully functioning, allow him to live with less stress and more in harmony. This has a direct effect on how the child reacts to his environment. If symptoms of dyslexia are reduced by these treatments it is because the child is less hypersensitive. It is a well-known fact that any form of stress tends to make a child's symptoms of dyslexia worse. Reducing that stress reduces the symptoms. But again, the underlying cause of the child's reactivity and sensitivity to stress has not been eliminated by these treatments. They do, however, have positive and beneficial effects on dyslexia and related conditions.

General body treatments

Acupuncture Acupuncture and acupressure for children usually produce a deep sense of relaxation. In children who are hyperactive, this may be a new feeling.

The majority of acupuncture treatments for children are painless and acupressure does not involve the use of needles at all. The instruments used on children are often special tools with blunt edges like the side of a large coin or a special little tapping mallet. Some are like small combs or gentle knobs. Tools of this sort may be used comfortably on infants as well as small children.

A typical one-hour session for a hyperactive child may involve only 5 minutes of treatment, given at 10- or 20-second intervals during the hour. The child is treated in the presence of the parent who holds or cuddles him while the gentle tapping is done. In general, children require much less treatment than adults and respond far more quickly. In older children (usually after seven years old) needles may be introduced. Acupuncture needles do not feel like injection needles and children soon learn that the sensation after acupuncture can be relaxing.

Educational kinesiology and 'Brain Gym' According to Paul Dennison, founder of educational kinesiology, or 'Edu-K', learning difficulties occur because of a lack of physical movement at crucial developmental stages. This can result in children getting confused and becoming unable to process information, or to participate in activities with others or manage their own behaviour. Stress also affects the way children move. Lack of integrated movement can lead to problems in writing and class participation. Problems in maths can come from a poorly developed sense of rhythm, sequence and timing.

The series of exercises called 'Brain Gym', which includes cross-body movements like skipping or crawling, trains the two halves of the brain to work in harmony. Well-developed use of the two eyes (binocular vision) is essential for successful reading, writing, and calculating. A child with poorly developed binocular skills will find it difficult to perform tasks such as catching a ball, reading aloud and copying from the board.

The above 'whole-body' treatments train the body to achieve balance and harmony and to reduce stress and blockages in energy flow. All these benefits will reduce levels of stress and thus levels of dyslexic symptoms.

Physiological causes

Treatments for physiological conditions

Megavitamin and trace element therapy High doses of specially chosen vitamins and minerals can produce changes in a child's mood (particularly depression that dyslexic children are prone to) and improve his ability to concentrate and study. The most commonly used are the Vitamin B complex vitamins. Different children respond to different vitamins so this type of treatment should be supervised by a trained nutritional therapist.

A controlled diet Treating symptoms of dyslexia by controlling what a child does and does not eat is becoming more widely recognized, along with a growing awareness of the many sub-stances in our modern environment which children can be hypersensitive to and which can cause negative symptoms. The list of substances known to have an adverse effect on a child's mental and emotional wellbeing include: processed foods, moulds, pollens, chemicals and food additives, antibiotics, chemical pollutants, and foods which have been sprayed with pesticides.

The increase in the incidence of dyslexia in children is more and more attributed to the decrease in the quality of their environment, poor nutrition and nutritional deficiencies.

Allergies and the Elimination Diet   Many common food substances – such as milk, wheat, eggs, corn and citrus fruit – are capable of causing an allergic reaction in children. If a child is suffering from allergies this can also negatively affect his ability to learn and study effectively and can have a marked effect on his ability to stay attentive and keep his energy in balance.

The Elimination Diet is a simple and direct way of discovering which particular antigens are causing reactions. The child is placed on a restricted diet, eliminating all the suspected foods that could be possible sources of allergic reactions. After about three weeks on this special diet, if there are noticeable improve-ments in the child's health, the child is given deliberate 'challenges' by adding back into the diet individual foods or additives to ascertain if noticeable side-effects return. Foods that cause reactions are removed from the diet. Care must be taken to ensure that restricted diets contain adequate amounts of protein, vitamins and minerals.

Again, reducing your child's emotional and physical stress levels will help to ease his dyslexic symptoms.

Behavioural causes

It is quite common that a child with learning difficulties will also have difficulties maintaining what is considered to be a normal profile of behaviours and attitudes. The most frequent behavioural and emotional symptoms associated with dyslexia are frustration and reactions to that frustration in the form of either rebellion or withdrawal. In addition, there may be present the range of symptoms commonly referred to as Attention Deficit Disorder, with or without hyperactivity. Problems can also be associated with a child feeling bad about himself and making assumptions about himself based on his capacity to perform. Lastly, a child who is constantly afraid of failing and not keeping up with his friends in school will be anxious and often depressed and unable to participate fully in a happy life at home and at school.

These behaviours are not technically symptoms of dyslexia. However, they are so much part of the whole picture of what it feels and looks like to be dyslexic that it is difficult to say just how much the learning difficulty is caused by malfunctions of the brain or sense organs and how much it is caused by disturbed behaviours that interfere with the learning process of the child. Consequently more and more attention is being given to a group of treatments for dyslexic children that deals with behavioural problems rather than the learning problems themselves.

Before starting any treatment for behaviours or emotions that may be shown by a dyslexic child it is important to determine how this set of behaviours is connected to his dyslexic symptoms. There are two possible connections:

1 The behavioural symptoms may be causing symptoms of the learning difficulty but are themselves the result of a different cause.
2 The behaviours are the result of secondary *reactions* to an underlying learning disability.

The classic example of the second possibility is the well-known 'class clown' syndrome. Here a child acts inappropriately in class and at home only as a way of defending himself from negative attention or negative feelings caused by being unable to learn like his friends.

When considering offering a child treatment for behaviours or emotions it is very important to be as clear as possible which of the above two relationships applies. In the second case, to address only the clowning behaviour of a child without also looking at the underlying cause – the learning disability – would be to preclude any real success when undergoing behavioural therapy.

Behaviours and emotions associated with dyslexia can be treated either psychologically or with medication. Psychological treatments fall into two categories, focusing on either the symptoms or the cause of the behaviours. Bach flower remedies may be used in conjunction with these or other therapies (*see* pages 62–3).

Psychological treatments for the behavioural symptoms

Counselling   In these treatments a child is given counselling in an attempt to give him behavioural skills to deal with situations where he has been behaving inappropriately or has inappropriate emotional reactions.

For parents of pre-school children and those just starting school, an early intervention programme will focus on the following:

- enriching the child's social and cognitive skills
- parenting skills
- increasing positive attention when the child is acting inappropriately or withdrawing
- using rewards
- developing effective discipline strategies
- using consequences
- using inductive reasoning

For a later age group (11–12 years and beyond), additional treatment could cover:

- dealing effectively with frustrated, aggressive, disruptive, oppositional and dysregulated behaviours
- dealing with withdrawal behaviours
- dealing with self-esteem issues and fear of failing

Biofeedback training   With biofeedback training a child can be taught how to consciously control the auto-nervous system through the use of biofeedback devices. Increasingly sophisticated biofeedback machines that use the power of computers can now map the activity of the brain waves and provide visual and auditory feedback to make the training more effective. In principle any negative symptom related to learning disabilities can be brought under control using these methods. Biofeedback is used not so much for changing actual perceptual abilities or processing abilities, but for alleviating psychological and emotional reactions to being learning disabled.

Counselling and biofeedback training are treatments for the symptoms of negative or disruptive behaviours. The underlying causes of such behaviours are not addressed by these approaches.

Psychological treatments for the causes of the behaviour
The two therapies described here are examples of therapies that work on the reduction of trauma. They have been used successfully with dyslexics to relieve them of the traumas associated with having a learning disability. The trauma is seen as the cause of the behaviours that produce symptoms of dyslexia.

Eye Movement Desensitization and Reprocessing (EMDR)   EMDR combines many elements from a range of therapeutic approaches with eye movements and other forms of rhythmical stimulation in order to stimulate the brain's information-processing system. This complex form of psychotherapy does not make use of past psychological material but instead activates the information-processing system of the brain so that recognizable and lasting changes are brought about in the fastest possible time.

Trauma Incident Reduction therapy (TIR)   TIR is a brief, one-on-one, non-hypnotic, simple and highly structured method for permanently eliminating the negative effects of past traumas. It involves repeated 'viewing' of a traumatic memory under conditions designed to enhance safety and minimize distractions. The client does all the work; the therapist or counsellor offers no interpretations or negative or positive evaluations, but gives only appropriate instructions to the client so that he can 'view' a traumatic incident thoroughly from beginning to end. A TIR session is not over until the client reaches an end point and feels good. This may take anywhere from a few minutes to 3–4 hours. An average session time for a new client is about 90 minutes.

Any psychological treatment that can help a child to be more emotionally in balance and free of fears and compulsions will obviously help in treating the real cause of the dyslexia.

Medication treatments   A growing number of therapists are recommending medication as a way of controlling and changing behaviours and associated emotions in learning disabled children. These drugs are most often prescribed for what is commonly known as Attention Deficit Disorder (ADD) or Attention Deficit Hyperactivity Disorder (ADHD).

A child with ADD will be unable to stay focused on a task for more than a few minutes, is easily distractible and unable to sit still for very long.

If hyperactivity is added to these basic symptoms the classification of ADHD is given. Associated with these primary symptoms will be a range of secondary symptoms which are often reactions to the negative attention drawn to a child who has these primary symptoms.

Stimulants   One of the known characteristics of dyslexic children is their abnormal reaction to certain medications, often the opposite of what would be expected in a non-dyslexic child.

Research some years ago into the effect of strong stimulants on dyslexic children found that instead of being stimulated by these drugs they were sedated. This information has been used to promote the idea that the negative behaviours of hyperactive children can be controlled by sedating them with stimulants.

Powerful stimulants such as methylphenidate (Ritalin), dextroamphetamine (Dexedrine) and pemoline (Cylert) are now available on the market and prescribed widely to children with symptoms of ADD and ADHD. There is no doubt that these drugs do modify their behaviour and remove the most disturbing symptoms. Children become quieter and more manageable and can concentrate on tasks for longer.

However, it is important to give a cautionary note on this particular form of therapy. If you are considering having a medication prescribed for your child it is always very important to find out as much as possible about any side-effects – especially of drugs as powerful as Ritalin and Cylert. Apart from any short-term side-effects, there is evidence to suggest that there are long-term side-effects that may have more serious negative consequences.

If the doctors offering or administering these drugs to your child do not have information on these side-effects, it is worth obtaining them from independent sources.

Medication treatments are the epitome of symptom-removal treatments for dyslexia. They do not in any way address the real underlying cause of the problems.

Bach flower remedies   These remedies, made from the extracts of plants and flowers, act as a catalyst to alleviate underlying emotional causes of stress and to establish equilibrium. They are non-interfering and thus may be used in conjunction with other treatments and therapies.

The flower essences are a perfect companion to any other form of treatment for children with learning disabilities. In some cases they may be all that is required. It is important to remember to look at the whole child when you are considering essences. A dyslexic child will often feel out of control and the essences can restore that feeling of control to him. The standard procedure is to treat a few symptoms initially and then gradually address the others. As the child begins to experience success he will feel more in control of his life. It is in this manner that essences can help. They may be given to the youngest children since they are harmless and have no side-effects.

Again, these flower remedies are used to alleviate symptoms without addressing the underlying cause. However, they are benign and do not have the serious side-effects that the stimulant drugs have on a child.

■ THE WAY FORWARD

It is helpful if parents can provide a long-term view of the future for their child rather than living on short-term solutions to immediate problems. By encouraging a dyslexic child to continue with his education or consider further treatment, parents can offer him continuity, structure and a perspective.

■ Leaving school and home

Continuity and structure are important for children as they face the prospect of moving out into the adult world. Some children may be so afraid of losing the known, familiar, protected environments of school and family that leaving home feels like falling off the edge of the world and disappearing.

Once your child has left school, there are many services and support facilities that he can take advantage of if he wants to go on with his education. Many colleges now have specially trained staff who can offer advice on vocational and career training as well as specific help with studying if needed.

A child's feeling of self-worth, self-esteem and self-confidence will determine greatly what doors are open to him as he leaves school or college and enters the job market and independent life. Whatever you can do to direct him into areas where he is able to use his natural abilities and talents will obviously help this transition to independence.

A dyslexic child leaving home can also be a difficult and daunting process for parents. After years dedicated to helping a learning disabled child, it can be a painful break to have to release him and trust his own resourcefulness.

■ Facing the future

Young adults' reactions to being learning disabled as they move out into the world can vary a great deal. Some of the more common reactions are:

- wanting to hide the fact of being disabled by over-achievement in work, sport or social relationships
- being afraid and unsure and feeling incapable of finding a place for themselves in the adult world of work and social relationships
- hiding by withdrawing and fading into the background of society, doing a job that does not challenge their talents and potential
- accepting the status of being disabled and making use of this status to find a place in society where dyslexics are accepted and accommodated
- becoming rebellious and non-cooperative and running the risk of clashing with law enforcement services
- giving up any attempt to integrate with social norms and expectations; exploring alternative lifestyles or allowing self-destructive use of drugs or alcohol to interfere with positive life choices
- looking for strongly structured environments or social groups or jobs – ranging from some of the more fundamentalist religious organizations to less benign groups that require

unquestioning allegiance – where they can feel safe and accepted if they accept the group's norms

A child needs to find a way to come to terms with whatever limitations remain after treatment in the areas affected by his disability. This process of acceptance and accommodation can vary tremendously from one child to another. Parents too must undergo this process. Your role has to be played with sensitivity and understanding at this point in your child's life. All pressure and explicit directives and attempts to control your child's choices should be avoided, however difficult that might be.

Sometimes parents are surprised by unexpected reactions, mood swings or uncharacteristic behaviour in their dyslexic child who apparently has made a successful integration into life and who is to all intents and purposes happy and successful. These sudden departures from normal or eruptions of emotion are signs that a dyslexic person can still be carrying his disability as a private burden and pain, despite all seeming to be well on the surface.

■ CONCLUSION

This chapter on the Orthodox Model of Dyslexia has described the many practical things that can be done to help a dyslexic child and the various treatments that can help to relieve his symptoms. But nowhere in this Orthodox Model is the fundamental cause of the dyslexia addressed or eliminated.

In the following chapter you can find out about the Davis Model of Dyslexia and how this does explain the real cause of dyslexia. You can also discover how dyslexic symptoms can be eliminated to the point where a child no longer has a learning disability.

3

The Davis Model

■ DEFINITIONS AND HISTORY

To correct dyslexia effectively we have to remove the actual cause of the dyslexic symptoms. When the cause is removed, the obstructions to learning are removed and learning can take place easily and naturally. Correcting dyslexia is not a matter of teaching a child how to learn. It is much more a question of removing what is preventing her natural ability to learn. When this is done properly a dyslexic child will learn quickly and thoroughly, and enjoy doing so. This may sound like a wild dream if you are a parent suffering with your dyslexic child's difficulties and frustrations. But thousands of children and adults have been able to remove their obstacles to learning and go on to learn whatever, wherever and whenever they choose. Using the Davis Model of Dyslexia they have been able to take control of their learning process.

■ A new meaning of dyslexia

The history of the word dyslexia in the Davis Model starts in the year 1980 in California. Ron Davis made his discovery about his own dyslexia when he was 38 years old. He had had severe learning difficulties at school and had been labelled uneducatably mentally retarded when he was a young boy.

His mother had been told by the doctors that he had a birth

defect called 'Kanner's Syndrome'. He had been told by doctors that he was unable to read or speak or remember his own name because his brain had been damaged during the birth process.

As he grew older Ron Davis was quite prepared to believe that what the doctors had told him was true. He had been unable to learn anything at school and even as an adult could not read a menu in a restaurant or a sign in a shop window. What the average person could read in five minutes or less took him an hour or more.

Despite his severe handicaps, like other dyslexics who want to hide their disability behind success, he became a certified mechanical engineer. At one point he owned and ran three engineering companies simultaneously. Later he moved to California and became so successful as a real estate agent that he retired at the age of 38 and took up his favourite hobby, sculpture.

While working on a sculpture one day he noticed something about his dyslexia that made no sense to the engineer in him. He noticed that if, while doing his sculpting, he tried to write notes, his handwriting was much worse than usual. It was quite bad anyway but when he was being creative with a sculpture it became impossible for even him to read. He had always been told that his bad handwriting was a symptom of his brain damage. That was the meaning of dyslexia he had been brought up to believe. But here he saw his symptoms changing – one minute they were worse and then later better again. As an engineer he knew that was not possible. If an engine is broken one day it cannot work the next day and then be broken the day after. If the structure of the brain is damaged the symptoms of that damage should always be the same. But he saw that one of his symptoms – his bad handwriting – changed depending on what he happened to be doing. His understanding of dyslexia as brain damage did not match the fact that his symptoms were changing without the structure being changed.

Perhaps if Ron Davis had been a person who thought with words rather than with pictures of meanings he would have ignored the changes that took place in his handwriting. But luckily for us all, Ron Davis thinks in pictures. His meaning of dyslexia suddenly had to expand to try and accommodate the interesting new facts about his handwriting. He became curious. He knew that when he was sculpting, his symptoms were worse, and when he stopped they improved again. Perhaps there was something else he could do to make the symptoms go away altogether?

Sure enough, after three days of trial and error with different ways of using his perceptual abilities, Ron Davis was able to go to a library and sit down and read *Treasure Island* from cover to cover in one day. He had never been able to read a book in his life before that day. He had had such difficulty reading that if he wanted to read a street sign he would have to stop the car and spell out the letters on it in order to read the name.

By expanding the meaning of what dyslexia is, Ron Davis found a way to understand what was causing his own dyslexia. With that understanding he was able turn off the dyslexia symptoms – and to turn them off so dramatically that he could suddenly read a book in one day. So he knew he had stumbled onto something. But he made an understandable mistake at that point. He thought he had cured himself of his learning difficulties. But this was not so. This expanded meaning of dyslexia was not quite big enough and did not yet contain all the ingredients necessary for a full understanding of how dyslexia happens and how it can be corrected.

A few months after his initial happy discovery, that he could read, Ron Davis' dyslexia symptoms started coming back. It was at that point that he began his search to expand the meaning of dyslexia even further until it completely matched the reality of what was happening to him.

With the help of a group of doctors, psychologists and educationists, Ron Davis set up the Reading Research Council in California. With his team he set about finding out what makes someone produce the symptoms of dyslexia. Ron Davis himself was the primary test subject for many of the experiments. Finally, after another two years, a new picture of dyslexia had been constructed. Once that picture was in place, it was clear what had to be done to prevent the symptoms of dyslexia. A way had been found to treat the real cause of dyslexia and eliminate it altogether.

■ The three ingredients

Ron Davis and his team of researchers found that dyslexia has three main ingredients. They discovered that for someone to be dyslexic three things had to be present:

- a certain way of thinking (picture thinking)
- a natural perceptual talent (ability to actively disorient)
- a specific way of reacting to confusion

These three things, in and of themselves, seem harmless enough. It is difficult to imagine how they could be responsible for all the problems dyslexics experience. But, working together, these three ingredients are responsible for all the symptoms of dyslexia and many other conditions associated with it. Such things as clumsiness, no sense of time, difficulty doing maths, hyperactivity and difficulty paying attention could all be traced back to these three ingredients working together to produce dyslexia.

What Ron Davis was able to do was find a picture of dyslexia into which you could fit all the very different symptoms of dyslexia. With this one picture it became possible to explain how all dyslexic symptoms develop from a single cause.

■ Disorientation

The key to the puzzle that he and his researchers found was a condition called 'disorientation'. Everyone knows what disorientation feels like – you lose the sense of where you are in relation to everything around you, you feel confused and unsure, you are not able to function normally. A very simple example is when you get dizzy, or when you wake up in a strange place and everything is unfamiliar. In fact when you are disoriented you will be confused about one or more of three things:

- the environment
- the identity of things
- time

When you are disoriented and confused you are much more likely to make mistakes. Mistakes with letters or numbers, mistakes in recognizing or saying words, mistakes in judging balance, distance and timing are all common of dyslexia. We could just as well call them symptoms of being disoriented and confused.

Removing disorientation

And now we begin to see how powerful this new picture of dyslexia can be in helping to correct the symptoms. If disorientation is the cause of the symptoms of dyslexia then by removing disorientation we should be able to remove the symptoms.

We all know how to remove certain kinds of disorientation. If you are dizzy you sit down and wait till your head clears and the world stops spinning around. If you wake up in a strange place you have to pause to remember where you are and then things start making sense again. Could it be possible that correcting dyslexia was as simple as removing the causes of disorientation? Ron Davis and his team of researchers found out that this was in fact the case. They found that dyslexic people are very sensitive to confusion and their natural reaction to confusion is to become disoriented. When disoriented they make the mistakes that we all call the symptoms of dyslexia.

The team at the Reading Research Council discovered that it was possible to teach dyslexics how to turn off the disorientations that caused them to make mistakes. An adult dyslexic could be shown how to turn off her disorientations and half an hour later read out of a newspaper for the first time in her life. When a dyslexic person experiences this sudden ability to read it feels as though some miracle has happened. But all that has

really happened is that the confusions caused by being disoriented have been removed. When a person is oriented, just as
you are as you read this book, that person is able to see accurately
and recognize words and read them. Being able to turn off
disorientation and stop confusion, however, does not mean
someone has been cured of dyslexia. That is only the first step
in the correction process.

Disorientation does not just happen to someone. Something
always causes it in the first place. You get dizzy when you spin
around too fast, for example. So in order to correct dyslexia,
something has to be done about what was causing the disorientations in the first place. Again, with the help of his team of
researchers, Ron Davis was able to describe exactly what was
needed to remove the causes of disorientation that dyslexics
react to.

What causes disorientation?

In the textbooks of psychology the symptoms of disorientation
are called 'beta apparent phenomena'. In layman's language this
means that sometimes our brains will make up things that are
only apparently there. We have a tendency to do this when we
need to make sense of what is going on around us.

If our eyes are telling us one thing but our sense of balance
and movement is saying something different, then conflicting
messages are going to our brain. Our brains do not like conflicting messages but are sophisticated enough to make sense of
the conflicting information we receive through our different
senses. But they do this by distorting our perceptions to achieve
a compromise. A specific function of the brain actually distorts
our perceptions in certain moments and makes us disoriented!
Disorientation is caused by confusion.

Making the connection

Ron Davis was able to make a connection between the brain's ability to cause disorientation and a particular talent that dyslexics have – a natural ability to see things in their imaginations very easily and vividly. Dyslexics can think in pictures very quickly and creatively, using three dimensions and movement – thinking with all their senses, in fact. It became clear that their ability to think in this way was causing them to disorient far more often than non-dyslexic people. In fact the symptoms of dyslexia, which are the symptoms made by someone who is disoriented, can be directly attributed to the dyslexic's talent to think in this special way.

To put it rather bluntly and crudely, it seems that dyslexics make their own dyslexic symptoms by doing something that they are good at. If they were aware they were causing themselves problems by thinking in this way, dyslexics would obviously not want to do so. But, unfortunately, this method of thinking and brain functioning is completely unconscious in dyslexics. Their talent is such an integral part of the way they think and see things that they use it automatically.

Ron Davis was not, in fact, the only person to make the connection between picture thinking and dyslexia. Thomas West, in his book *In the Mind's Eye*, describes the lives of a number of highly successful creative geniuses, such as Leonardo da Vinci, Thomas Edison, Nikola Tesla and Winston Churchill. All these remarkable people had many of the symptoms of dyslexia as children, and some even as adults. And a remarkable woman, Nel Ojemann working in Holland, had made the connection between picture thinking and learning difficulties forty years before Ron Davis stumbled upon his own understanding of how dyslexics create their dyslexic symptoms.

▓ Correcting the dyslexia

What Ron Davis and his team of co-workers did was to take the understanding of what causes dyslexia and produce a treatment that successfully removes this cause. The treatment process for a dyslexic child involves a few simple steps:

1 helping her to become aware of how her natural talent is being used
2 helping her to understand and be aware of how this natural talent can cause disorientation and subsequently confusion and mistakes
3 teaching her the practical things she can do, based on this understanding, to remove the confusion from symbols (usually words) that cause her to disorient

These simple steps make up the basis of the Davis treatment for dyslexia, a programme that has helped thousands of dyslexics to overcome their learning difficulties.

▓ The real cause of learning difficulties

Ron Davis' picture for dyslexia needed one more dimension to make it an effective tool for correcting dyslexia. Up until now we have been talking about the more mechanical processes of dyslexia. We have seen how the dyslexic's perceptual talent can actually cause disorientation and confusion because of inaccurate perceptions. Add the dimension of 'trying to learn' to these confusions and we begin to see the full picture of how a learning difficulty develops. The following scenario is typical for a child with learning difficulties.

1 The child is trying to learn something.
2 Because she is confused, she becomes disoriented.
3 When disoriented her senses are distorted.
4 Distorted senses mean she receives inaccurate information.
5 While disoriented she is trying to learn things with this inaccurate information. She is therefore learning the wrong information.

6 She then has to reproduce what she has learnt. The information comes out wrong because it went in wrong. The wrong information she gives out is called a mistake by the teacher.

7 She becomes more and more frustrated with her mistakes because she cannot see why she is making them. She cannot see that the information she is taking in is wrong before she even begins to try and reproduce it.

The emotion that comes with this dilemma, of getting information that is already wrong, is frustration. If you were to ask 100 dyslexics what is the emotion they most associate with their dyslexia, probably 95 per cent would reply 'frustration'.

Dyslexia is more than just a mechanical process in the brain. The true picture of dyslexia is one of someone trying to cope with living in a confusing world, making mistakes, not knowing why she is making those mistakes and trying to survive. This is why dyslexia for each child is different because each child has different ways of making mistakes and finds different ways to cope and survive.

■ Dealing with frustration

A dyslexic child at some point will become so frustrated by the mistakes she is making that she will start to find ways to get over, round or under her feelings of frustration in order not to be overwhelmed by them. Usually this starts to happen with a child at about the age of 8–9 years old.

Each dyslexic child will begin to develop her own set of solutions for dealing with her frustration. Whatever form these solutions take they will have all something in common.

1 They will be certain ways of doing things and tactics for knowing and remembering things.

2 They will have worked at least once before being adopted.

3 They are roundabout methods for coping with the effects of disorientations and the mistakes that are made as a result.

The solutions will become compulsive behaviours – the only way a child can do something in a particular situation. Most children will at some point stop using the alphabet song because they have learnt the sequence of letters correctly, but for a dyslexic who is using the alphabet song as a way of remembering, it will be a compulsive behaviour. The child will have to sing that song every time she wants to look up a word in the dictionary and she will not be able to stop doing this however hard she tries.

■ The true obstruction to the learning process

The problem with these compulsive behaviour solutions is that they interfere with the learning process. They become the only way a child can perform a certain function. It is these behaviours, in fact, that create the learning disability.

The mistakes made as a result of disorientations are not the true learning disability. All of us make mistakes as part of a learning process. The disability stems from the limitations imposed on the learning process when a child is compelled to behave in certain ways in reaction to confusions. Therefore the only way to correct the learning disability in a dyslexic child is to dismantle and remove these compulsive behaviours, the obstacles to real learning. Again, through more experiments and research, Ron Davis and the Reading Research Council team were able to understand how this could be done. Once the obstructions are removed the real learning process can begin to take place and the difficulties with learning seem to evaporate. More about compulsive behaviours and how they can be overcome will be found in the Treatment section beginning on page 112.

■ A guided tour of dyslexia

To add more details to the Davis Model of dyslexia, this section is presented in the form of a guided tour through a theme park where you are able to experience things first hand. I hope it brings across something of the feeling given to dyslexia by Ron Davis' approach. It is certainly very different from the feeling you get from the Orthodox Model.

When you first enter the exhibition area of this imaginary theme park you are greeted by a group of dyslexic children ranging in age from 8 to 16, your tour guides. If you can relax and let them lead you through the various exhibits you should have some fun and learn about another way of looking at dyslexia.

Exhibit I: Picture and Word Thinking Show

Peter is the first to come up to you and grab your hand. He says excitedly, 'Come over here and see how we think!' You are dragged into a nearby sound booth with a large screen at the other end. Peter pushes you in and slams the door shut before switching on some equipment. Words move across the screen. They form a simple story about a boy taking a dog for a walk in the woods. As you see the words, a voice reads them out over loudspeakers. Peter opens the door and comes back in.

'Got the idea?' he asks. 'This is called word thinking. When you do it you hear the sounds of words in your head. We don't. Dyslexics don't think with the sounds of words.'

You are then moved hastily out and into an adjacent booth. Again the door is slammed shut by Peter and he goes over to a film projector and switches on. You recognize the same story but this time there are no words. Just a silent film, in colour, of a boy taking his dog for a walk in the woods.

'Listen!' says Peter, in a dramatic stage whisper. 'That's what it sounds like when I think. I just see the pictures. No sound in my head! This is what we do when we think. OK. That's enough. Let's go on!' and he races out of the booth and round to the next corner.

'Hang on, you guys!' you say. 'Let me get this straight before we go on. Are you saying that dyslexics think in pictures and other people think in sounds? Like when I talk to myself when trying to park the car?'

'Exactly!' all the children shout in unison.

'But what does that mean?' you ask, as it is not quite clear.

'It means,' says Simon, with exaggerated patience, 'that it is very difficult for me to learn any word if you give me the sound first. I have to have a picture in my mind of what the word means and then if you tell me the sound I can remember it much better. So I can't learn words by breaking them up into pieces of sound. I get really confused. And then I just get frustrated because I can't understand what is being said. And I stop hearing after a while. I just hear bits and pieces. And then if I still have to sit there I go off.'

'Where do you go?' you ask, curious about what Simon does when he is bored.

'I just go off and think about something else I like. It's what happens. I can't stop myself and then I don't even hear what you are saying to me.'

'OK,' you say. 'I've got it. What's next?'

Exhibit II: The Perceptual Talent Machine

Simon has now joined Peter and they are standing proudly in front of a huge whirlygig machine, just like the ones in fairgrounds where you sit in little capsules on the end of long arms and are whirled and whizzed around at frightening speed.

'Get in and hold on tight,' they say.

The boys clamber into one of the capsules after you and sit down at a control panel. Before you have even got a chance to get comfortable the whirlygig is off on its mad ride. The two boys next to you are as cool as cucumbers, steering the capsule in all sorts of complicated manoeuvres.

'OK, time to stop!' you manage to yell after a while and they reluctantly bring the capsule back down to the ground.

'So what was all that meant to show me about dyslexics?' you ask.

'OK,' says Peter, refusing to come out straight and tell you. 'Now close your eyes and imagine the house where you live. Tell me when you can see a picture of where you live. Can you see it?'

You nod your head when you have a picture of your home in mind.

'Right,' says Simon, taking up the interrogation, 'what do you see? Tell me what part of your house you are looking at in your picture.'

'The front,' you say.

'Are you standing at the front gate or are you by the front door?' Simon continues.

'I'm looking at my house from the front gate,' you tell him.

'Good, open your eyes. That's it,' he says. 'That is all this machine is.'

'Oh? Tell me more.'

'OK. You were standing looking at the picture of your house in your imagination from the front gate.'

'Yes,' you reply.

'Well, that's our talent. That place where you were standing looking at your house . . . we call that place something.'

'Mind's eye!' shouts out Angela. 'That's what we call the place we look from when we look at the imaginary pictures in our mind.'

'OK,' you say. 'So what about this mind's eye?'

'Dyslexics have something we call our Perceptual Talent. We can move our mind's eye and put it in different places to look at the pictures in our imagination. Just like we did in the whirlygig machine, our mind's eye can go around and up and down looking at the pictures we make in our minds.'

'But our mind's eye goes much much faster than that,' says Angela.

'And are you all good at it?' you ask.

'Yes,' all the children shout out.

'So why do you move your mind's eye around so much?' you continue.

'We look at things from all directions – up, down, from the side. Very fast. I can see the other side of the whirlygig in my imagination, by looking at it with my mind's eye. It's easy. We start doing it when we are really young.'

'I do it without thinking about it,' says Peter. 'In class I do it quite a lot. When the teacher is boring. I know what is going on everywhere. Even outside the class and behind me. I just use my mind's eye to see what is going on. I get distracted a lot. I also know exactly what the teacher is feeling. And the other boys in my class. I just know somehow. I can feel it.'

'Yeah. I just go off and watch the pictures in my mind when I can't do the sums on the blackboard. Trouble is I can't hear what the teacher is saying when I'm doing that,' adds Simon.

'Why can't you hear the teacher when you are moving your mind's eye?' you ask.

'We get disoriented when we move our mind's eye.'

'Disoriented? What does that mean?' you ask.

'It means we are not seeing what our eyes really see and not hearing what our ears are really hearing. We are confused by what is going on around us,' says Simon.

The other children join in.

'And we don't know if time is going fast or slow.'

'And we can feel like we are moving when actually we are sitting still.'

'Everything gets confusing when we are moving our mind's eye around.'

'I can't see the words on the page that I am reading when I am disoriented,' says Judy.

'I feel dizzy,' Peter adds. 'And if it's really bad I feel like I'm going to be sick.'

'I find it helps to tap on the floor when I'm reading. It stops me feeling so dizzy. That is also disorientation. It comes from reading and writing. I get it when I am trying to do joined up letters. Then it's bad.' This is Angela talking.

'I get so confused then I make mistakes and the teacher gets so cross with me and everyone laughs. I hate it,' Judy adds.

'So what you are all saying is that when you move your mind's eye you get disoriented, and then you feel confused and even dizzy. And then you make mistakes. Is that right?' you ask.

'Yes! Well done!' The children congratulate you for getting the point they are making so quickly.

Now Simon is pushing you across to a live demonstration of the third characteristic that all dyslexics have.

Exhibit III: The Threshold for Confusion

'OK, stand just here,' Peter instructs. 'On this spot. Don't move and don't look up.' He is quite insistent so you obediently stand still on the spot and wait rather nervously. You know something is about to happen but are not quite sure what. Above and in front of you is a big container on pivots. It is slowly being tipped towards you by Simon who is winding a handle. You can now see that it is filled almost to the brim with hundreds of coloured ping-pong balls. Peter is standing on a raised platform pouring more buckets of balls into the container as it slowly tips towards you. The container is delicately balanced now. You can see that if Peter throws in one more bucketful the whole thing will tip over and you will be hit by an avalanche of ping-pong balls. And of course that is exactly what happens.

'Yeahh!' shout all the children together, fully enjoying the sight of you submerged under the ping-pong balls.

'And what is all that meant to show me?' you ask.

'That is the third thing that dyslexics have that other people don't,' shouts down Peter. 'Those balls are the confusion and we are very sensitive to confusion.'

'I can tell you what it is like,' says Angela. 'I'll be doing something at school. Some exercise. And then it gets harder and harder but I keep going and get confused. Then I get so confused that my mind's eye moves and I'm disoriented. That makes me even more confused. It's like that container. I just get to a point where it's too much. Off I go.'

'Off you go, where?' you ask.

'When the confusion gets too much my mind's eye just takes off and I'm disoriented. I just want to get away. Sometimes I just have to get up and walk away somewhere else. If I'm not allowed to move, my mind's eye goes off somewhere. I disorient.'

'When that last bucket went in,' says Peter, 'that's when the container tipped. We call that point the threshold. When we get too much confusion we go over the threshold and get disoriented.'

'And dyslexics are special,' adds Judy. 'We have quite a small container. Not like that big one. I get confused really quickly.'

'We have a low threshold,' says Angela. 'Other people who are not dyslexic last longer before they get confused. We tip over much sooner.'

'That's because we have a mind's eye that moves. Normally we don't get confused much outside. I know most of the time what's going on. It's only when I'm in class and reading or something. Then I get confused, by words and things, and numbers and what the teacher says. Then I can't work it out and get confused and then it all just gets too much.'

'Can you tell me a bit more what it is like being disoriented?' you ask.

'Don't worry,' says Simon. 'Not everyone can understand how this works the first time. Dyslexics usually understand it straight away but others need more time. You see, it is not something strange that only dyslexics do. Everybody does it sometimes. Come over here and stand by this bench.'

You follow his instructions. Simon sits on the bench and you stand in front of him.

'Now, turn round ten times as fast as you can and then sit down here next to me,' he says.

You dutifully spin around ten times and clumsily sit next to Simon as fast as you can, your head spinning. He hands you a sheet of paper, and asks, 'What does this say?'

You look at the sheet and can see there are words written there, but they are blurry and swimming around. 'I can't tell. Everything is spinning around.'

The children call out 'Sound it out!', 'Try harder!'

'What do you feel?' asks Simon.

'Like I'm just about to fall off the end of the bench,' you groan.

'Good. End of demonstration,' says Simon. 'That's what we mean when we say that our brain makes up things that are not actually going on when we move our mind's eye. We call it disorientation. Just like what happened to you after you had spun around. I knew the world was not actually moving and that the words were clear, because I was not disoriented. You felt you were going to fall over. But I could see you were sitting still. So it happens to everybody sometimes. The same thing happens when you are in a train and the train next to you in the station starts to move but you think you are moving. Your eyes are telling you one thing – that you are moving forwards – but your stomach knows that you are not moving. Because this does not make sense to your brain, it makes you feel like you are moving when you are not.

'Dyslexic children are different from other children because we do it a lot more than just once in a while. Whenever we are confused by something we move our mind's eye to try and work out what it is we are seeing. So whenever we are confused our brain starts to make up what it thinks we *should* be seeing and hearing and feeling. We get disoriented and things are different for us than for everyone else. We go in and out of it. Sometimes it is just for a short time. Other times we can be disoriented for an hour or more. We also get disoriented when we are day dreaming. The same thing is happening but it is our mind's eye that moves.

'When we are disoriented we can't hear properly what the teacher or mum or dad is saying to us. We can't see clearly what is on the board and we can't follow instructions. We are confused by all sorts of other things around us. It gets very frustrating.'

'OK, thanks. I've got it. What's next?' you ask.

Exhibit IV: The Back-to-Front Bicycle

Sally hands me a bicycle saying, 'Just ride this bicycle down to that tree and back. It's quite easy.'

You clamber on obediently and as soon as you start pedalling you know you are in for a fall. It is one of those trick bicycles where you have to turn the handlebars the opposite way than you would normally do to stay in balance. After trying for a few minutes and getting only a few feet down the path, with several ignominious falls on the way, you give up. You are boiling with frustration and feeling like a fool in front of all the watching children. They can see from your face that you have got the point.

Angela speaks up. 'We just wanted to show you what it is like when parents or teachers treat us as though we cannot look after ourselves. We aren't stupid and helpless'.

'Are you starting to get more of an idea of how it works for dyslexics?' Peter asks.

Exhibit V: The Gemstone Model

Sally beckons you over to a low building with a darkened entrance, in a garden with a large sign on the door stating 'The Gemstone of Dyslexia'. You walk together into a large dimly-lit room. All that is in the room is a large gemstone, perhaps 2 feet across. As you walk closer you see it is just a hologram hanging there in mid-air. As you look closer you can see deeper into the gem. Below the surface of each facet there are pictures of people doing things. As you walk around admiring it Simon runs up and says, 'Look, I've got this one, this one and this one over here.' He runs around pointing to different facets on the gemstone.

'What do you mean?' you ask.

'Well, each of these places represents a different thing that dyslexics can do. Some of them are good things – like I am very good at drawing and I can play soccer for my school. And some of them are bad things – like here is bad at reading and here is no good at handwriting and this one is can't add up. So they are all mixed up together, good ones next to bad ones.'

'So you mean people can have a mixture of good and bad at the same time?' You ask.

'Of course,' Simon says. 'That's what it's like being dyslexic. There was someone here yesterday who had nearly all good things, but he was still wetting his bed. That's on here too somewhere.'

'Are you telling me that dyslexia is not just the things you find difficult but also the things you are better at than other children?'

'Yes, of course!' shout all the children at once. 'That's why some people say you have the *Gift* of Dyslexia.'

Exhibit VI: The Three Pillars

Before you know it you are standing in front of three enormous white pillars at the top of a hill. Resting on the capstone above the pillars is the word DISORIENTATION cut out in huge letters. Carved into the capstone itself are the words CON-FUSION ABOUT. And each of the three pillars has a name carved into it:

ENVIRONMENT
IDENTITY
TIME

'What does confusion about environment mean?' you ask.

'That's when I don't know where I am. Don't know left from right. What is up or down, things like that. Can't follow things along one after the other.'

'What about identity?'

'Simple. That's when I look at something and I have no idea. I look at a letter or a word and it's just blank. Identity is what something is. It's when you look at something or hear something and you don't know what it means.'

'And time?'

'That's obvious isn't it. You know when you don't know how long it takes to do something or what time it is and can't tell time on a clock. It doesn't mean anything to me.'

Oscar pipes in, he is only about eight or nine. 'I never used to know if breakfast came after supper of before. I didn't know what was going to happen when I came home from school. I was happy at school because I was told what to do next. But in the afternoon after school I didn't. I got afraid because I never knew what to do with myself.'

'And you know now?'

'Yes. Listen!' And he tells you the sequence of meal times in his day.

Exhibit VII: The Garden of Symbols

Now the children all rush off to a small garden. You are led over to one side where, standing in the middle of a circular lawn, is a tree. The lawn is surrounded and divided in half by a low box hedge. Standing by the tree is the word TREE in 3-foot-high polystyrene letters. On the other side of the lawn is a head, also made out of polystyrene, with its mouth open. Oscar reaches up and yanks on the ear lobe of the head. The mouth slowly opens and a loud mechanical voice announces 'TREE'.

'That is a symbol!' say the children together triumphantly.

'Explain it to me,' you say. 'I haven't quite got it.'

'A symbol has three parts – what it means, what it looks like and what it sounds like,' the children chant in unison.

You still look confused so the children chant again and as each part of the symbol is named one of them runs up and touches the relevant part of the symbol on the lawn – first the tree, then the large letters and last of all the head making the sound.

'OK,' you say, 'now I get it. So the tree in the middle is what the symbol means and the other two are the sound and the sight symbols.'

'Yes, that's right. We are picture thinkers. So we go straight to the middle first and then we can add on the two other parts.'

The children now lead you to another circular lawn in the garden, also divided in half by a box hedge. On the left are three 3-foot-high polystyrene letters – T H E. On the right is another large head. Judy runs up to the head, pulls the ear and the sound of 'THE' comes booming out. But in the middle space between the letters and the sound there is nothing on the grass, just an empty space.

'So where is the meaning?' you ask the children, looking round.

'You tell us,' they laugh knowingly. 'You tell us what "the" means.'

For a moment your mind goes blank.

'Too late, too late,' the children all call out, dancing around you.

'What do you mean, too late?' you ask.

'When we are reading and we see a word we don't know the meaning of, we just get confused. If we get a lot of words with nothing in the middle, like this word "the", we have so many blank pictures in our thinking that we get too confused. Our mind's eye starts to move about.'

'And then what happens?' you ask.

'We get disoriented. And then we start making mistakes,' replies Peter. 'When I'm standing up in class trying to read and I get one of these blank words where there is no meaning I get confused and my mind's eye moves. I miss the next word or say it wrong and everyone laughs. That makes everything worse. I lose it all then and have no idea what I'm doing. It's terrible. But that's what used to happen. Now I can read without those blank pictures.'

'How can you do that?' you ask, intrigued.

Peter says, 'I'll show you,' and walks over to a white plank on the lawn and steps on it. A section of the lawn opens up and a statue of a boy pointing to a ball at his feet, rises up. The statue announces 'The ball! That one which is here or which has been mentioned'.

Peter turns to you and says, 'You have just discovered the meaning of "the". We have to add the meaning! We think with the meaning of the words, that is the most important part for us.'

Finally, seeing the logic of it, you ask, 'How do you do that? How do you add the meaning?'

'Wait, we'll tell you. But first you have to come and see our special movie theatre over here.'

Exhibit VIII: The Blank Picture Movie

You are ushered into a small movie theatre and Judy turns on the projector. A man is talking about the words that dyslexics find hard to read because their meaning is difficult to understand.

'There are more than 200 of these words,' Angela confides to me. 'I have done 26 so far. They are all the silly little words like "and" and "to" and "on" and "once" – the sorts of words that we are meant to remember but can't because we have nothing to remember them by.'

'We call them our "trigger words",' adds Oscar.

Suddenly the screen goes blank and the sound goes off – just for a moment. And then the film resumes, but you have difficulty picking up the story again. Just as you feel you have caught up, the screen goes blank again, this time for a longer period. When the picture finally returns you have lost the point of the story. The film then rewinds to the beginning and starts to play through again. But the same thing happens at the same places. You leave the film studio in frustration.

'So tell me what you were trying to show me in there.'

'The blank picture comes when we read the trigger word,' says Judy. 'When we get too many in something we are reading then we get so confused. Then our mind's eye moves around to try and get rid of the confusion. When that happens we stop seeing what is really in the book. Our brains start to make up things or miss things out. Then we have to try going back and starting again to make sense of it. But the same thing happens. I just used to give up after a while. I could never get to the end and make any sense of it. I got a headache when I read because of those trigger words. I had to concentrate so hard.'

As you are talking the children are leading you towards a large glass building in the park. Finally you ask the most important question, 'But what can you do about it?'

Peter points at the building and says, 'This!'

Inside the building you can see children and adults sitting at tables. On the tables are books that look like dictionaries, and people are making things out of clay. Each person is making something different.

'What are they doing?' you ask.

Judy says, 'They are mastering their triggers!'

Peter adds, 'They are oriented and they are creating the meanings of the words in clay models so that they can think with them. That stops the blank pictures happening.'

Finally all of the pieces have come together. 'It's really that simple?' you ask.

The children giggle and smile in agreement.

'And it's easy!' adds Judy. 'We use the way we think to add meaning to the words. Learning is easy, if we're taught in the same way that we think!'

■ Your tour guides

There are a few things that are immediately obvious about the children that have been showing you around the Davis Theme Park of Dyslexia.

1 They are self-confident and self-assured. They feel sure of what they are telling you about because it is coming from their own direct experience. The meaning of their experiences fits the meanings in the Davis Model of dyslexia.

2 They talk about their learning difficulties in a different way than

you would expect. It is obvious that the children understand what is happening when they have difficulties at school. And they feel that they are able to correct these difficulties with their understanding about how their dyslexia works. They are already busy using the tools given to them by this new understanding and relating to their environment with this new point of view.

■ HELPING YOUR CHILD

For a deeper understanding of how the parts of dyslexia work together it is best to refer to Ron Davis' own books about dyslexia (*see* Further Reading). But I hope you now have a sufficiently clear picture of what can be happening with your dyslexic child so that you may be able to help her, using this model.

Obviously the ideal situation would be one where your child also has an understanding of how her dyslexia is working. If she can understand what is happening to her when she gets overwhelmed by confusion and when she becomes disoriented, she can understand why she makes the mistakes she does. She can also understand what she has to do to turn off these disorientations and to stop making mistakes.

What I can give here are some general guidelines for helping your child. If you understand the underlying principles on which these guidelines are based then you can apply them to your own family situation. This means that instead of having a huge book of rules to follow, you can adapt what you know to fit your own particular child and family needs.

What you can do to help depends primarily on the age of your child. I have divided this section into four different age groups. The divisions themselves represent the ages at which there tend to be significant developments or changes in a child's dyslexia.

1 Up to age 6
2 From 6 to 9

3 From 9 to 12
4 Beyond age 12

In each part there are references to the three basic concepts described in the guided tour of the theme park of dyslexia. These concepts can help in explaining why a child is showing a certain set of symptoms. They can also explain what is the best action to take in response to these symptoms.

As a reminder, the concepts referred to are outlined below.

Basic concepts

Picture thinking

One of the most important things to understand about your child's dyslexia is that it is something that develops and changes as she grows. This progression is directly connected with another development that happens in all children as they grow up – the way in which they think. As mentioned earlier, there are two primary ways of thinking – either in pictures, using meanings or ideas and concepts; or in words, using the sounds of words, as though you are having a conversation inside your head.

All children, before they are able to use and think with words, are picture thinkers. The age at which a child starts to use word thinking as well as picture thinking has a direct effect on the development of dyslexic symptoms.

For a child to show the most commonly recognized symptoms of dyslexia she has to be primarily a picture thinker up until the age of nine. Most children after the age of about five are able to think in both words and pictures. What makes dyslexic children different from other children is that they develop word thinking much later.

Almost all of the learning a child is required to do at school needs word thinking. Any child who is primarily a picture thinker will have difficulty learning information that is presented primarily in the form of sounds. Sounds do not always have meanings attached and this is what makes it so difficult for the picture-thinking child who needs the meaning of a word to make sense of the information.

Some dyslexic children will hardly ever think in words. It is these children who will have the most difficulty at school and in any environment where words and sounds are the primary form of communication.

The threshold for confusion

Dyslexic children are more sensitive to confusion. The point at which they experience being overwhelmed by confusion we can call the 'threshold for confusion'. Dyslexic children have a lower threshold. This threshold or sensitivity is not static or fixed. It moves up and down, even in the course of a day.

Besides confusion about words and symbols there are other factors that can lower the threshold and affect a child's ability to maintain orientation. This list compiled by the Reading Research Council can help you to become aware of what can make your child's dyslexic symptoms worse:

- insufficient rest
- poor diet or not enough food
- illness, pain or injury
- drugs or medicines
- very small print
- very faint print
- varying print styles and typefaces
- loud noises
- specific sounds
- certain smells
- poor lighting (too much or too little)
- excess motion (whirling fans, dangling decorations)
- rearranged furniture
- change in the orderliness of the environment
- moving house

- unscheduled changes
- threats of punishment
- family strife
- fear
- loss
- anything that is a reminder of a past unpleasant experience

Disorientation

The talent to move the mind's eye, and thus disorient and alter sensory perceptions, is active in dyslexic children. These disorientations and subsequent distortions of perception can take place as a reaction to confusion about three factors: the environment, the identity of something, and time. Disorientations may also occur when dyslexic children fantasize and day-dream. During these activities the brain functions in the same way as it does when they are reacting to confusion. This means the same distortions of perceptions will be present.

1 Up to age 6

In a child of this age we are not looking for a learning disability. We are looking for two characteristics: is the child a picture thinker, and does she have the talent for moving the mind's eye?

Signs to watch out for

- Take into account that dyslexic children are never average. They will never be 'somewhere in the middle' of any range of possibilities. They will always be found at the extremes of any scale. A dyslexic child may be very slow to walk or talk, but on the other hand she could be walking or talking in full sentences long before what would be considered 'normal'.

- Bear in mind also that all symptoms of the learning disability may be symptoms of something else rather than reactions to confusion. Apparent impairments in any of the senses – sight, hearing, balance and coordination – should obviously be medically checked if they persist. Should the tests prove that your child has nothing wrong with her senses then you can suspect that her impairments and learning difficulties may be caused by disorientations as a result of confusion or day-dreaming.
- If the child shows an interest in playing with clay this activity can be included as part of a preparation for going to school. Making the letters of the alphabet in clay together with your child, without any pressure or expectations being placed upon her, will give her direct experience of the symbols she will meet in school.
- If you notice that your child becomes confused in certain situations or environments be aware of the effect this will have on her senses. She may become disoriented and not hear what you are saying. She may also become clumsy and unco-ordinated and break and drop things.
- If your child is day-dreaming a lot it should be taken into account. This will affect her ability to develop an inherent sense of time. She may have more difficulties with sequence and order than other children.
- Remember the 'Gemstone Model' of dyslexia and be on the lookout for the talents your child has, even at this early age. Do not just concentrate on the things she might be having difficulty with. Emphasize and encourage her talents and this will give her a solid base on which to build on when it is time to start working with symbols and other confusions she may be having.
- If your child has started at kindergarten you may be getting reports back from the teacher that do not match what you know your child to be like. Don't be concerned or upset with the teacher, or surprised. It may be that when your child is at home she is not demonstrating any of the symptoms of dyslexia. At school there may be more confusions and other

factors that lower her threshold for confusion so that symptoms of dyslexia may be appearing there that you do not see at home. Just the stress and emotion of being at school can be enough to lower the threshold and cause dyslexic symptoms and the associated reactions to appear.

■ 2 From 6 to 9

Signs to watch out for

- particular difficulty learning to read and write
- persistent and continued reversing of numbers and letters (eg '15' for '51', 'b' for 'd')
- difficulty telling left from right
- difficulty learning the alphabet and multiplication tables, and remembering sequences such as the days of the week and months of the year
- continued difficulty with tying shoelaces, ball-catching, skipping, etc
- inattention and poor concentration
- frustration, possibly leading to behavioural problems

General points to consider

- Your child may have been coping up to a certain point at school then suddenly seems to reach a barrier that is too much for her. Usually the barrier is about having to work with symbols which are confusing.
- Signs of rebellion or withdrawal in your child indicate that she has reached this barrier of confusion and frustration and cannot get past it in school work.
- Look for signs of dwindling self-esteem, self-doubt, crises with her friends at school, not feeling good enough, self-inflicted withdrawal from her friends.
- Short attention span when doing a task is a sign that something is confusing your child. When she gets to a point of

confusion and frustration because she cannot understand something, she will be overwhelmed by confusion and have to withdraw by going away. This going away may seem as though she cannot keep her attention on one thing for very long. If she understood what it was she was meant to do and was not confused she would have no problem focusing on the task. For most children, computer games are a good example of something that holds their attention and at which they can succeed.

- If you give instructions to your child and she does not appear to be listening or does not carry out what you asked her to do, very likely this is due to some confusion that has caused a disorientation. Once this happens she will not be able to hear what you say accurately because she is disoriented. Look for this 'not listening' symptom before deciding it is just bad behaviour or poor memory.

- Is your child working extremely hard preparing for tests but still getting most of it wrong? She may appear to be stupid and not understanding but it is likely that confusion with symbols is the problem. The stress of taking a test will also lower her threshold for confusion. This makes it even more likely that she will be disoriented during the test itself and thus will not perform to the best of her ability.

What you can do?

This is the age group where intervention with treatment for learning difficulties is most important. The actual techniques for this intervention are described in the Treatment section (*see* page 112). The Release Procedure described on pages 26–8 is a very practical way to help a child who gets tired, tense and nervous about producing school work on time and doing tests.

Awareness of the problem   Before the age of seven a child is probably not fully aware of having a problem that is serious enough to be treated. She may be coping and getting along to some degree. It is only when she hits her first real barrier to learning that she will be motivated enough to do something about her difficulties. The frustration she feels at making so many mistakes has to reach a certain level before she will be ready to do something about her problems.

At age eight or nine a child would be ready to learn about controlling her disorientations using training in the Davis methods (*see* Treatment section). This will help her with turning off the distortions in perceptions which occur whenever a confusion triggers disorientation. She would also be able to learn about mastering the confusing symbols that are the real cause of her difficulties and frustrations (see pages 118–21).

Starting early   If the training with orientation and work with symbol mastery can begin soon enough, a child may avoid the added problem of developing a set of compulsive behaviours in response to the frustration of making mistakes.

The other advantage of beginning the correction of the dyslexia at this point is that there are fewer problems connected with a child's self-esteem and feelings of self-confidence. The longer a child struggles and fails at school, the lower her self-esteem will go. In addition, the behaviours of withdrawal or rebellion that she adopts in reaction to these emotions and the frustration that comes from failing, will be more developed.

Accommodating dyslexics in school   Schools and teachers have very differing opinions about how to accommodate the 10 per cent of children who each year fail to keep up with their peers. With education budgets severely restricted, any school proposing to give some of its pupils special, one-on-one attention has to justify this extra expense. So even if both parents and teacher agree that a child would benefit from extra classes to help with a learning disability, it may not be within a school's budget to provide this service.

■ 3 From 9 to 12

Signs to watch out for

The following descriptions of the symptoms of a child with dyslexia, caused by disorientation have been adapted from the list compiled by Alice Davis, Ron Davis' wife and a director of the Reading Research Council. It provides a useful summary of signs and symptoms.

General
1 Appears bright, highly intelligent and articulate but below average at reading, writing and spelling.
2 Labelled lazy, dumb, careless, immature, 'not trying hard enough'; has behaviour problems.
3 Is not sufficiently behind to be given extra help at school.
4 Has a high IQ but may not test well academically; tests well orally but not in written work.
5 Feels dumb; has poor self esteem; hides or covers up weaknesses with ingenious compensatory strategies; easily frustrated and emotional about school, reading or testing.
6 Talented in arts, drama, music, sports, mechanics, story-telling, sales, business, designing, building or engineering.
7 Seems to 'Zone out' or day-dream often; gets lost easily or loses track of time.
8 Has difficulty sustaining attention; a day-dreamer.
9 Learns best through hands-on experience, demonstrations, experimentation, observation and visual aids.

Vision, reading and spelling
1 Complains of dizziness, headaches or stomachaches while reading.
2 Confused by letters, numbers, words, sequences or verbal explanations.
3 In reading and/or writing makes repetitions, additions, transpositions, omissions, substitutions, and reversals in letters, numbers and/or words.

Distorted perceptions

1 Complains of feeling and seeing non-existent movement while reading, writing or copying.
2 Seems to have difficulty with vision, yet eye examination does not reveal any problem.
3 Extremely keen sighted and observant, or, at the other extreme, lacks depth perception and peripheral vision.
4 Reads and re-reads a text with little comprehension.
5 Spells phonetically and inconsistently.

Hearing and speech

1 Has extended hearing: hears things not said or apparent to others; easily distracted by sounds.
2 Finds difficulty putting thoughts into words; speaks in halting phrases; leaves sentences incomplete; stutters under stress; mispronounces long words or transposes phrases, words and syllables when speaking.

Writing and motor skills

1 Has trouble with writing or copying; pencil grip is unusual; handwriting varies or is illegible.
2 Clumsy, uncoordinated, poor at ball games or team sports; has difficulties with fine and/or gross motor skills and tasks; prone to motion sickness.
3 Can be ambidextrous, often confuses left/right, over/under.

Maths and time management

1 Has difficulty telling time, managing time, learning sequenced information and tasks or being on time.
2 In maths shows dependence on finger counting and other tricks; knows answers but cannot write them down.
3 Can count, but has difficulty counting objects and dealing with money.
4 Can do arithmetic, but fails word problems; cannot grasp algebra or higher maths.

Memory and cognition

1 Has excellent long-term memory for experiences, locations or faces; poor memory of sequences and unexperienced facts and information.

2 Thinks primarily with images and feelings, not with the sounds of words (little internal dialogue).

Behaviour, health, development and personality

1 Is either extremely disorderly or compulsively orderly.

2 Can be class clown, trouble maker, or too quiet.

3 Had unusually early or late developmental stages – talking, crawling, walking, tying shoe laces.

4 Is prone to ear infections, sensitive to foods, additives and chemical products.

5 Has an opposite reaction to medication than normal children – a sedative acts as a stimulant, the dosages required for a particular medication to have an effect are different from those given to normal children.

6 Can be an extra-deep or a light sleeper.

7 Wets the bed beyond appropriate age.

8 Has an unusually high or low tolerance to pain.

9 Has strong sense of justice, emotionally sensitive; strives for perfection.

10 Makes more mistakes and symptoms increase dramatically with confusion, time pressure, emotional stress and poor health.

Further signs

1 A child who has had no apparent problems at school in the first five years may suddenly meet a barrier that she cannot cross. It will represent a sudden stop in her progress through school.

2 Forms of rebellion – not wanting to go to school, not wanting to do school work – are signs of a reaction to the frustration of hitting a barrier at school that seems insurmountable.

3 A child may lie about school performance to avoid confrontation with failure.

4 Signs of an identity crisis in a child will indicate that the barrier mentioned above has been hit. She may start to think that she is stupid, whereas up until this point she had managed to convince herself that there was nothing wrong.

5 A child may give up and stop trying at school, a further sign that she is now finding the frustration of not being able to understand too much to cope with.

6 Specific signs may show up in a child's school work: handwriting may still not be cursive; adding, subtracting and multiplying may be manageable but division appears to be impossible.

7 Teachers may also start to become frustrated with the lack of progress in a child's school work, whereas before they were enthusiastic about finding other ways to help.

8 Parents may start to doubt that their child really is bright and intelligent. They are finding it difficult to go on convincing themselves of this.

What you can do

Here again, the most important help you can give a child of this age is to give her the ability to control her perceptions through the Davis treatment for dyslexia. You will also be able to help her, having done the initial Davis treatment programme, to work on removing the confusing symbols in her environment that are causing the disorientations.

If this Davis treatment is not immediately available to you from a trained Davis Dyslexia counsellor, you can offer the following practical help to your child:

- Help her to understand what is causing her frustration and why some symbols are confusing.
- Learn about and understand the threshold for confusion and discover with her what are the situations and conditions that lower her threshold (*see* pages 94–5).

- Inform the school about the cause of your child's difficulties and enlist teachers' support and help where possible.
- Find ways to reduce emotional stress and time pressure both at school and at home since they are major factors in lowering the threshold for confusion.
- Find areas where she can excel and build up her self-esteem and self-confidence.
- Never address her rebellion directly. It is more important to remove the cause of the rebellion. More often than not she is reacting to the frustration of not being able to keep up with the demands of school and feeling she is not good enough.

Beyond age 12

The next most common barrier met by school children with dyslexia occurs when they reach the age of 14 or 15. At this time in their school work they are required more and more to start applying the basic concepts and information they have learnt up to this point. A child may have managed to survive by means of rote learning and reciting parrot-fashion what she has heard, but she will not really have understood what she has memorized. Then, suddenly at 14–15 she is required to think with concepts and ideas and finds she cannot rely solely on her memory. When her memorization solutions no longer work it can feel like she has met a solid barrier, and one which she can do nothing about.

Because she is now older and more mature – both physically and emotionally – the reactions to the frustration of meeting this barrier are likely to be different and more extreme than those of a child between 9 and 12 years old. A violent or depressed 15-year-old has a far more severe problem than a younger child with the same feelings.

An added complication at this age is the onset of puberty. The ups and downs of hormonal and emotional changes affect a child's threshold for confusion. This leads to more frequent episodes of disorientation and the consequent effect of making mistakes, being confused and feeling frustrated at not under-standing what is needed.

This is the most critical period in a dyslexic child's life. The stage is being set at this age for her future relationship with herself and with society. A child at this point really has to find a way to establish and maintain some form of self-esteem and self-worth. If not she may well have difficulties in the future, turning to crime even or experiencing mental problems. A study made of a penal institution in the United States revealed that 98 per cent of the inmates had learning problems. Confrontation with the law is an almost inevitable future for someone who feels frustrated and less worthy than others.

Signs to watch out for

- serious problems with self-esteem
- physical violence or verbal abuse as part of the expression of rebellion
- clashes with the law – getting into trouble
- mixing with the wrong friends
- experimenting with alcohol and drugs
- increased moodiness, with mood swings
- rebellion now expressed at home as well as at school
- truancy from school; refusal to do school work
- laziness, not caring any more
- no longer trying
- extreme withdrawal rather than rebellion; possible suicide attempts

What you can do

As with the previous two age groups, the most essential help for a child of this age is to give her a way of understanding and using her natural talents. Rebuilding her feelings of self-worth and self-confidence are much more important than how much learning is going on in the classroom. The fundamental attitude of a child has to be established before any learning can be resumed.

Learning to control her orientation and learning to use symbol mastery (*see* pages 118–21) to deal with the confusing symbols and concepts in her environment will help to remove the frustration. She will start to realize that she is not stupid and incapable. Removing the frustration starts to remove all the reactions that grow from that frustration.

At this age it may be more difficult for a child to accept help from parents. She may be so far into her rebellion and non-cooperation that anything her parents offer is rejected as a matter of principle. In these situations there may be a way for someone she trusts and respects, who is not part of the family, to bring her the message that there is a solution. In the end there is no way parents can force their child to accept the help offered in the form of the Davis correction methods for dyslexia. It is sometimes very difficult for parents to have to accept this. A child's dyslexia can be corrected only if she herself wants to be helped.

■ HELPING YOURSELF

Many of the suggestions given in the Helping Yourself section of the Orthodox Model (*see* pages 31–41) also apply in this approach to dyslexia. The crucial difference with the Davis approach is that it does not see dyslexia as an incurable disability. In this model it is not seen as something that has to be coped with, adapted to and accepted. Dyslexia is the Gemstone that can be a mixture of both talents and difficulties.

With the Davis Model, parents have a very different role to play when helping their child. Below I have listed some key points to get you started on helping yourself. It is not a comprehensive list but is enough to give you a feel of how the meaning of dyslexia given in the Davis Model can be used to guide you. There is no particular sequence to this list.

■ Let go of concern

Parents of dyslexic children may suggest that it is impossible to find the space and time for themselves because their lives are organized around the needs of their dyslexic child. This way of living is often a result of their concern and worry about their dyslexic child and her future.

Concern, worry and anxiety are the things that parents find most difficult to shut off. These feelings tend to seep through any barriers you try and construct. A common example makes the point. You have arranged for your child to spend a few days away with your own parents in order to have some precious days on your own, but what do you find yourself doing? Worrying about your child and her future and feeling guilty perhaps that you are not doing more to find a solution to her problem!

I hope this book will enable you to start letting go of that concern and worry. Its message is truly this:

• There is nothing to worry about.
• There is nothing fundamentally wrong with your child.
• Your child's dyslexia can be corrected.

■ Eliminate confusion

Eliminate as much confusion – mental, emotional and physical – from your child's environment as possible. Try to keep an orderly environment at all levels. And help your child to do the same. (See 'Threshold for confusion' on pages 94–5.)

It is very important not to give confusing and conflicting messages. As far as possible, what you say and what you are doing and feeling should be coherent and consistent. Practise being certain and clear in all communications and decisions you take regarding your dyslexic child.

■ Create a feeling of certainty

One of the primary needs of a dyslexic child is a feeling of certainty. If she is certain about something she can relax. Uncertainty will make her lose whatever self-confidence she may have managed to build up.

■ Remember picture thinking

A simple thing to remember here is that your dyslexic child, being a picture thinker, has very clear pictures in her imagination of things that you tell her and things that she is expecting to happen. If circumstances, for whatever reason, change and things do not happen in the way she was expecting them to happen, her pictures of how it should be are in conflict with reality. Her pictures are just as real as what everyone else sees. It is sometimes very hard for her to let go of these pictures and accept something else.

A simple example. You are about to take your child on a trip in the car. In a moment, without thinking, you have promised her that she can sit in the front with you. At the last moment someone else decides to come with you and she ends up having to sit in the back. What should have been an enjoyable and exciting adventure turns out to be a nightmare. She is upset and angry and you cannot understand why. What has happened is that your daughter's picture of the trip, sitting in the front of the car, has not happened. It is almost impossible for her to let go of that picture and be with the reality of the moment. She is very disappointed, way beyond what you might have expected.

This is just a way of saying that it is important to be careful about what you promise your child. Once what you have promised becomes a picture, any change will be difficult for her to manage.

When a dyslexic child lacks certainty in herself she will automatically look to her parents for that need. If she cannot find it there her threshold of confusion will be low and she will more readily be confused and disoriented.

■ Be a haven of safety

In the normal non-dyslexic world a dyslexic child's identity is under continual attack. Because of her difficulties in learning and in school work she will receive more criticism and negative attention than other children. She will be trying as hard as she can to establish an identity that is acceptable at school and yet everything seems to fail. In this desperate situation she needs unconditional love and acceptance from her parents, far more than other children.

■ Do not allow school to invade your home

If a child finds at home more of the same expectations and non-acceptance that she has encountered at school, her world and identity are threatened on all sides. She will feel that there is no longer any safe place where she can just be who she is. She will not have anywhere to relax, a place where she does not have to try to be someone that she cannot be.

It is a very common assumption and belief amongst parents that they should present to their child the same point of view that the school presents during the day, so that expectations and demands are consistent at both home and school. Children who are able to keep up with their work and meet the expectations of school will have no problem with this. With the dyslexic child there is a difference. Parents who uphold the school's demands and expectations only make their child's suffering worse rather than increase her ability to develop self-responsibility and self-discipline, which was their intention. This is not to say that no demands or expectations should be made of a dyslexic child. But any demand or expectation should be within the context of unconditional acceptance and love.

It is often quite difficult for parents to make and maintain this distinction and home becomes an extension of school. The pressures on parents from school and other social forces – both explicit and implicit – can sometimes be more than they can resist. And yet a dyslexic child needs to know that whatever she does and however it turns out she will still be loved and accepted for who she is.

■ TESTING

One of the main purposes of conducting tests for dyslexia is to find out to what degree some activity differs from a chosen norm – how many mistakes a child makes or how far away she is from some chosen ideal.

When you know your child is dyslexic then the details of the symptoms of her dyslexia are not so important. What is more important is removing the *cause* of those symptoms. When the cause is removed the symptoms will no longer appear.

With the Davis Model the emphasis or direction of testing is thus changed from symptoms to causes. This makes testing for dyslexia very simple. It involves finding out if a child is able to think in pictures and has the natural talent to move her mind's eye and become disoriented in the process.

■ What the Davis test will tell you

The test will not tell you if your child is dyslexic. It will simply tell you that *if* her symptoms are caused by these two character-istics (thinking in pictures and being able to move her mind's eye) then she can be helped to learn how to control the conse-quent disorientations and turn them on and off as needed. She can thus be shown how to correct her symptoms of dyslexia. The test takes about 30 minutes to perform and if the results show that she is able to think in pictures and move her mind's eye then the indications are that she could benefit from the Davis Dyslexia Correction Programme – if she has the motivation to do so. A full description of the test procedure can be found in Ron Davis' book, *The Gift of Dyslexia*. He has written the instructions in such a way that parents can test their own children. If you do not feel confident to carry out this test on your child it can be done by another adult whom she trusts or by a trained Davis counsellor.

■ When paediatric testing is needed

If the symptoms of dyslexia are not caused by these two charac-teristics, other factors, such as deficiencies in the physical sense organs, might be responsible. The standard paediatric testing described in the Orthodox Model chapter (*see* pages 20–1) would therefore apply in these cases.

There is a rare dyslexic condition which does not fit into this general model. It occurs when a child adopts an 'old solution' which prevents her visualizing and/or moving her mind's eye. A child with this sort of dyslexia should be referred to a Davis Dyslexia Correction specialist for help.

■ The Point of Intervention

The moment when testing is done depends a great deal on the development of the child. Testing according to the Orthodox Model is normally done before about the age of seven or eight. A younger child may show signs of disorientation but not yet have any learning difficulties. The frustration of making mistakes and not being able to keep up in class will eventually reach a point where the child is motivated to do something about her dyslexia. That is the best time to introduce the idea of doing a test and to start helping her understand what is going on with her orientation and perceptions. Before that time she may not be too interested in controlling her disorientations because they have not yet become a sufficient problem for her to want to do things differently.

On the other hand, testing according to the Davis Model of

dyslexia is simple, quick and fun to do and in no way demands that a child perform or be judged according to some set of standards. In this sense, because the test is not implying that there is something wrong with the child, the Point of Intervention is not so critical.

■ TREATMENT

The Davis Model of treatment for dyslexia is designed to remove the *cause* of the symptoms. The symptoms themselves are not treated directly.

The Davis Treatment Programme comprises the following steps.

■ 1 Establishing a Symptom Profile

Once a child has been tested to find out if she has the two characteristics of dyslexia – an ability to think in pictures and a natural talent of being able to actively move the mind's eye – the next step before any actual training takes place is to create an individual Symptom Profile for the child. This will give the Davis counsellor a picture of what ingredients are present in that particular child's form of dyslexia.

The reason for doing this is that children have different ways of being disoriented and coping with the difficulties that creates. Every child has a different set of factors that affects the threshold for confusion. No two dyslexics have exactly the same set of symptoms. A training programme for correcting a child's dyslexia therefore needs to be designed specifically for that child. Because the basic Davis Treatment Programme is adjusted to meet individual needs, there is no standard Davis Treatment Programme for all dyslexics, although the basic ingredients are the same in each treatment. How those ingredients are combined and which ones are given emphasis depends entirely on the needs of the child being treated.

To give a feeling for how and why a Symptom Profile is

compiled we might slip back for a moment to the Guided Tour of the Davis Theme Park of Dyslexia. We will ask our group of dyslexic children to explain how they created their own Symptom Profiles.

Exhibit IX: The Avenue of My Dyslexia

The children invite you to walk with them down The Avenue of My Dyslexia. At the entrance to the avenue of tall trees a man is standing by a stall with huge bunches of red and white balloons. Each child is given a bunch and they set off running down the avenue. They stop and fix a balloon on each tree trunk – at various heights.

'What on earth are you doing?' you ask Simon.

'Well, the red ones represent what we are good at and they go on one side of the avenue, the white balloons go on the other side for things we are not so good at. The trees are the different sorts of things we do – there is a reading tree, a spelling tree, a football tree, even a tree for how we get on with our parents! The high balloons mean you are really, really good at something. Peter has put his red balloon high up on the music tree because he plays the trumpet really well. By the time you get to the end of the avenue you can look back and see what you are good at as well as where you don't do so well.'

You then understand that each child can see at a glance how his or her dyslexia is a balance of talents and difficulties.

At the end of the avenue there is a wishing well and a basket of shiny coins to throw in to it.

'What happens here?' you ask.

'We make a wish for what we would like to be better at after doing a training programme for dyslexia,' says Simon. 'I'm going to throw in three coins because I want to be able to read better, to be able to play tennis with mum, and to have more friends at school.'

You thank the children for showing you their Avenues of Dyslexia.

The Avenue of My Dyslexia highlights several points about creating a child's Symptom Profile:

- It establishes a child's strengths as well as weaknesses.
- It allows a child to evaluate herself in a number of different areas.
- It is carried out in a non-threatening and supportive manner that will be continued on into the training.
- It can be used to cross-check a child's sense of herself and to pick up any divergence between what the parent sees and what the child sees.
- It provides a useful tool for designing a tailor-made treatment for the specific needs of a child.
- The wishing well is designed to show that it is important that a child's perceived needs are met. If a child is put through a programme to improve her reading but actually what she is more concerned about is her maths then the programme will not be so effective.
- The child's motivation and interest and enthusiasm for doing a Correction Programme are the prerequisites for beginning treatment in the Davis Model approach.

The most commonly treated symptoms

Below are the most commonly treated symptoms of dyslexia that can be reduced or eliminated by the Davis Treatment Programme.

Confusion about identity of symbols (words and letters)

Reading
- slow reading – anywhere from a third to one tenth the speed of a normal reader
- low reading stamina – not enjoying reading, getting tired easily
- re-reading text many times in order to understand

Spelling
- letter reversal problems
- letter order
- remembering a word one day but not the next

Handwriting
- badly formed letters
- writing not following horizontal
- pressing pen too hard on paper or holding pen too tightly

Speech difficulties
- inability to reproduce a sound that is spoken
- inability to hear certain sounds
- problems with pronunciation

Punctuation marks
- not seeing punctuation marks when reading
- not knowing what punctuation marks are used for

Capitalization
- not understanding how capitalization is used

Using a dictionary
- inability to look up words because of difficulty with sequence of letters in alphabet

Confusion about numbers
- not knowing the meaning of numerals and their relationship to numbers

Confusion about the physical environment

Dyspraxia
- poor coordination, clumsiness
- inability to walk up and down stairs easily or stand on one foot

- difficulty catching balls
- proneness to accidents, frequently bumping into things or knocking things over
- inability to cross mid-line of body, difficulty with tying shoe laces
- confusion between left and right
- letter and number reversals – turning letters and numbers upside down or back to front
- bedwetting – the child is confused, thinking she is *actually* in the bathroom or toilet when she wets her bed, when in fact she is still asleep in bed

Confusion about time

- inability to estimate passage of time
- inability to tell time on a clock

Confusion about sequence

- inability to put things in sequence
- problems with spelling
- problems with arithmetic
- missed out letters and numbers
- not understanding the concept of sequence
- difficulty with days of the week and months of the year, sequence of daily activities
- difficulty with counting, adding
- difficulty with following a set of instructions
- letter and number reversals – putting the letters or numbers in the wrong order within a word or number

Confusion about order and disorder

- difficulty with maths
- difficulty with organizing environments, thoughts, actions
- difficulty with paying attention

Attention Deficit Disorder and hyperactivity

There is one set of conditions caused by a combination of confusions about environment, identity and time that is commonly known as ADD or ADHD (*see* page 61).

Phobias

The set of symptoms called phobias also have disorientation as their underlying cause.

Based on the understanding of what is causing a child's learning difficulty, the treatment can be very simple and straightforward. The two main goals of any treatment according to the Davis Model, called Davis Orientation Counselling, are covered in steps 2 and 3.

▨ 2 Davis Orientation Counselling

In Davis Orientation Counselling a child is taught how to control the disorientations that result from confusion. First of all she must be able to detect when she is disoriented. Then she must be able to turn the disorientations off. The symptoms of dyslexia are simply the symptoms of disorientation. By turning off the disorientations she is in effect turning off the symptoms of dyslexia.

A child is able to turn off her disorientations by learning how to orient her mind's eye in relation to a point in space behind and above her head. The simple fact of having her mind's eye in a particular position relative to her body has the effect of disengaging the function of the brain that causes the disorientation and the altered perceptions that accompany it.

Once a child has experienced what it feels like to be oriented she can more easily notice the difference between this feeling and the feeling of being disoriented. Being oriented feels a lot more comfortable than being disoriented and confused. Once they are oriented accurately, dyslexics often speak of being in a 'comfort zone'. They sense a whole-body feeling of wellbeing and being connected to the earth, and are more at rest and ease.

Each dyslexic person will have different sensations and perceptions to identify the difference between being oriented and disoriented. Some of the commonest experiences associated with becoming disoriented are:

- feelings of dizziness or falling
- feelings of confusion, blurred vision, distorted sounds
- feelings of uncertainty and clumsiness
- making mistakes and misjudging distances
- words moving on the paper
- moving out of the 'comfort zone'

The initial session of Davis Orientation Counselling usually lasts less than an hour. At the end of the session, if it is successful, the child will be able to become orientated by intentionally positioning her mind's eye at a particular 'orientation point'. She will be able to re-orient herself easily and quickly, and know when she has done it. As a result of being oriented her reading skill may improve appreciably, even after this one initial session.

Although the sudden ability to turn off the symptoms of dyslexia may seem like a dramatic cure for dyslexia, this is not really the case. The cause of the *symptoms* – the disorientations – might have been removed, but this is only the first step in the Correction Programme. The following step – the removal of the cause of the *disorientations* – is just as important.

■ 3 Symbol Mastery

Removing the cause of the disorientations is where the real work of correcting dyslexia begins.

The things that cause disorientation in a dyslexic child are the things she finds confusing. It might be a letter, a word, a sound, an idea, or even time itself. The name given in the Davis Model to all these 'confusion-causing items' is 'triggers'. A trigger is anything that is sufficiently confusing to cause the dyslexic persons minds eye to move away from its 'orientation point.' But a child will not be able to start on this next step of the Correction Programme unless she has the correct perceptions that come with being oriented. A more detailed description of this process is given in Ron Davis' book *The Gift of Dyslexia*.

Removing the triggers

How can a trigger be made inactive so that it is no longer capable of causing disorientations and confusion? The process is simple in principle, although slightly more complex in execution. By removing the confusing element from any symbol it ceases to be a trigger and becomes just like any other symbol, something that means or is a representation of something else.

The process used to remove confusion from a symbol is called 'Symbol Mastery'. 'Mastery' is the process of learning something so well that you can do it without thinking about what you are doing, riding a bicycle, for example. But to master something you first have to acquire the necessary knowledge and experience of that thing. When you master something you become certain. So to master a trigger symbol you have to take the confusion out of that symbol and stop it causing a disorientation. This can be done with triggers such as letters, punctuation marks, numerals, sounds and words. In fact, all the most common symbols that cause confusion for dyslexics and thus trigger the disorientations can be mastered using this technique.

How is a symbol mastered?

By creating the meaning of a symbol in the form of a clay model we create our knowledge of that meaning in our experience. That is all we need to do to master the meaning of a word or symbol that is causing confusion.

A simple example may make it clearer. A common trigger

word for dyslexics is, surprisingly, the word 'in'. If you look at the meaning of this word in a dictionary you will find quite a few different meanings. Mastery of a word using clay goes through a number of steps:

1 Take just one of these meanings from the dictionary, for example 'to the inside of'.

2 Make sure your child is clear about this meaning and has a clear picture of it.

3 Make a model of the meaning in clay. It could perhaps be of a hand placing a bunch of flowers in a vase. It can be that simple.

4 Place beside this model of the meaning a model of what the word looks like in letters.

5 The next step is to connect the sound of the word 'in' to the models. By saying the word 'in' while making a mental picture of both the clay model of the meaning and the letters, your child will have mastered the symbol of the word 'in'.

6 The confusion about the picture that goes with the word 'in' will be removed.

7 The word 'in' will have been mastered and will no longer be a trigger word.

Once a symbol is mastered a child can think with that symbol in pictures. For a dyslexic child who thinks in pictures, it is filling in the blank pictures were causing the confusion (*see* Exhibit VIII 'The Blank Picture Movie House') . Once the blank pictures are filled in using Symbol Mastery the confusions no longer occur and the disorientations are not triggered. Without disorientations a child's perceptions remain accurate and con-sistent and she can see the words on the page clearly and learn to read them.

It sounds very simple, almost too simple to be true. How could something that has such a dramatic effect on a child's ability to read be learnt in a matter of hours?

The Davis treatment does not try to teach children something that is strange and unfamiliar. It is helping them to control a talent they already have. All dyslexic children have the ability to turn disorientations on and off. All that has been missing up to this point is that they have never been shown how to *control* that natural ability.

Teaching a child to do this can be likened to teaching a child who is naturally musical how to control her ability to play a musical instrument. Once a child knows how to control her disorientations and can do so quickly and easily, and knows when she has done so, the Orientation counselling will have been successful.

Creating clay models of the meanings of all the words and symbols that are triggers is not something that can be done in just a few hours. But by steady application and persistence any child can work through the triggering symbols and master them all. At that point it would be true to say that a child's dyslexia had been corrected. When all the trigger symbols are mastered, the child will be able to think with the meanings of those symbols and will not be confused by them.

■ 4 Treatments for specific difficulties

Spell Reading

Spell Reading was developed by Ron Davis at the Reading Research Council in the United States. It is very simple to use and very effective in helping children improve their reading skills. The system is based on Ron Davis' knowledge of how dyslexics tend to perceive things and how they need certainty in order to function effectively.

Before this Spell Reading system can achieve maximum effectiveness a child should have learnt how to control her orientation and, preferably, to have removed any confusions from the letter symbols of the alphabet. But the principles on which Spell Reading are based still work even if these prerequisites have not been fully met.

Principles   A dyslexic student's awareness tends to be spread out around the environment. When reading, a dyslexic child tends to look at a word on the page in the same way that she looks at the environment. She tends to take in the whole word at once rather than starting on the left and moving to the right.

This way of perceiving words tends to make the dyslexic guess at what she has seen because she is not looking in a way that will help her see the word accurately. When she starts to guess, any feeling of certainty goes away and it becomes very difficult for her to gain confidence in reading.

Spell Reading aims to train the dyslexic child to move her eyes from left to right when reading and to recognize letter groups as words, and to put the sound of the whole word together with the picture of the group of letters that make that word.

Procedures   In the first part of Spell Reading, a parent or counsellor sits with the child, takes a book and covers the text with two pieces of paper. One piece allows only one line at a time to be exposed and the other allows, as it is moved, only one letter of each word on that line to be exposed at a time. As the second piece of paper moves from left to right across the page, the child is asked to say the name of each letter as it is revealed.

The movement across the line trains the dyslexic child's eyes to look at a word from left to right. Most of us take it for granted that this is how to look at a word. For a dyslexic child this can be a new experience because she is used to looking at a word randomly from any direction.

This simple procedure is also used to help the child recognize the shape of a word – how the letters follow each other in a particular sequence, from left to right. The counsellor or parent also tells the child what a particular word sounds like so that she can learn to put a particular sound with a particular shape of letters and look at that shape from left to right. As the child gets better at moving her eyes from left to right and at recognizing which sounds go with which word, the pieces of paper covering the text can be removed. The child is then allowed to read the words by sweeping her finger along the line of text, uncovering one word at a time. This is further training in moving the eyes from left to right across the page and in seeing the letters of the words from left to right.

Up to this point the child is not expected to understand what she reads. It is purely an exercise in 'technical' reading – recognizing words and putting the right sound with each word. But she can be helped to understand by an additional procedure, Picture-at-Punctuation, which makes use of the dyslexic's ability to think in pictures. The child is asked to make a picture of each phrase in a sentence, using the punctuation marks as a way of dividing it up into natural pieces each with its own picture.

The 'Fine Tuning' procedure for clumsiness

For these symptoms to be fully corrected the Fine Tuning procedure is added to the Davis Dyslexia Correction Programme. The objective of this exercise is to find an orientation point for the mind's eye where the senses are most accurate and consistent, rather like turning the dial on an old-fashioned radio set until you find the best reception. As the mind's eye moves very slightly back and forth around the orientation point, the senses of balance and movement are used to tell when an optimum point is reached. Once established this optimum point can be checked in a very simple way. A child is asked to place her mind's eye on her optimum point and then balance on one foot. Two balls are then thrown towards the child, simultaneously, and she has to catch one in each hand without falling over. If she can do this it means that her senses of balance, timing and vision are accurate and she is using her optimum orientation point to achieve this.

For any child who has difficulties with coordination, catching two balls at the same time while standing on one foot would be an impossible task. Using her optimum orientation point, any child with dyspraxia caused by disorientation will be able to do this exercise, with a little practice, consistently and confidently. It is a very direct and effective way for a child to experience what a difference it makes to have her mind's eye located on the optimum orientation point.

This procedure is usually carried out on the third day of the five-day Davis Dyslexia Correction Programme.

Treatment for agraphia or dysgraphia (poor handwriting)

As mentioned earlier, poor handwriting can have a number of causes. If it is not a reaction to being unable to spell, it is usually due to the child having multiple pictures of what the letters should look like or perceptual problems when seeing certain forms or lines that are required in handwriting. Specific procedures can be used to help a child achieve clear, legible handwriting in a matter of hours.

The commonest cause of handwriting problems is that a child has been shown so many different ways of making letters that she has multiple mental pictures of how they should look. When she writes she is trying to write all these different pictures at the same time and ends up with a jumble of lines and letters that move all over the place. By helping the child to remove all the overlayed pictures of what letters should look like and to replace them with a single picture that is accurate, she can follow that picture and her handwriting will become clear and legible.

Some children write badly in order to cover up not being able to spell correctly. When this spelling improves, so does their handwriting.

Another possible cause comes from the fact that some children, due to their being disorientated a great deal, have not developed the ability to perceive certain shapes or lines. The necessary neural pathways in the brain, for instance, that allow us to see a diagonal line, will not develop in some children if their perceptions are often distorted by disorientations. When a child cannot see diagonal lines she will not be able to write any letters with these lines in them. Using orientation and with practice these neural pathways can be opened up and within a few days, with further instruction on how to write the shapes, letters can be formed normally.

Symbol Mastery of fundamental concepts

By mastering the meanings of the fundamental concepts of consequence, time, sequence, order and disorder, a child will begin to to think with the meanings of these concepts.

Mastery of a concept follows the same steps as mastery of a confusing symbol. An experience of the knowledge of a concept is created by making a clay model to represent the meaning of that concept. Once a dyslexic child has a clear picture of the meaning of a concept she can begin to think with that concept. For complete mastery of fundamental concepts such as time, sequence, order and disorder, a child must also be able to control her disorientations. By maintaining orientation she will begin to experience a consistent and accurate impression of her environment, perhaps for the very first time. These consistent and accurate perceptions provide a foundation on which the fundamental concepts can begin to be internalized and truly mastered.

Treatment without medication for Attention Deficit Disorder and hyperactivity

As mentioned in the Treatment section of the Orthodox Model (*see* pages 61–2), these conditions are conventionally treated using powerful stimulants such as Ritalin and Cylert to modify behaviour.

Because dyslexic children, when disoriented, can have an opposite reaction to medication than normal children, these stimulants have a subduing effect on them and are administered for this very reason. There have been serious doubts expressed by some researchers about the safety of these drugs, especially when administered over a long period of time.

Leaving aside the moral and ethical issues of whether medication should be administered to children to change their behaviour, the most important thing to know about both ADD and ADHD is that the primary symptoms are all symptoms of disorientation and confusion about a few fundamental concepts, and so can be treated and completely eliminated using the same Davis Dyslexia correction methods used for other learning disabilities. There is absolutely no need to use medication to treat these conditions.

Most people when referring to ADD and ADHD give more attention to the secondary symptoms of these conditions, which are often more dramatic and disturbing. The reactions of a dyslexic child to the frustration of not being able to perform simple tasks because of confusion and disorientation, when added to hyperactivity, can lead a child into a range of behaviours that is disturbing both for herself and for her classmates, teachers and parents.

Treatment for phobias

The difference between phobias and dyslexia is simply the source of the disorientation. In dyslexia the source of disorientation is *confusion* – about the environment, about the identity of things and about time. The source of disorientation for phobic symptoms is *fear*. It is important when trying to understand the cause of a child's dyslexic symptoms to make the distinction between these two sources of disorientation. It is possible, for instance, that if a child is showing acute symptoms of disorientation and confusion before or during tests or exams, the source of that disorientation could be the fear of failing at the exam rather than any confusion about symbols or words.

Whether a child is disorienting because of confusion or because of fear, the treatment involves teaching the child how to control her disorientation to the point where she can turn the confusions off.

The training for learning how to control disorientations caused by fear is different from the training for learning how to control disorientations caused by confusion. This is because the reactions of a person in response to fear are usually more powerful and disturbing than those of someone responding to confusion. The training to control orientation involves showing a child how she can repeatedly move from disorientation to orientation when exposed to a disorienting stimulus. When this technique is applied to phobic reactions, the child is exposed to the fear that is the cause of the disorientation. For this reason it is essential that orientation training to overcome a phobia should be carried out only by a professionally qualified Davis counsellor.

▓ 5 Assembling the tools to take home

The normal Davis Dyslexia Correction Programme is given over five consecutive days. It is a one-on-one programme – one child with a counsellor. In those five days the child is given a metaphorical 'box of tools' which will enable her to:

- understand what she needs to do to maintain or restore her orientation when required
- recognize when she is disoriented and what the triggers are that cause those disorientations
- understand how disorientation alters perceptions and makes learning much more difficult
- work with clay to eliminate confusion from trigger words
- relax and release the tension that comes from concentrating too hard on achieving a task
- control energy levels in her body so that she can adjust them to the appropriate level for any activity she is engaged in
- create certainty, which will increase her self-confidence
- possess a set of fundamental principles that she can think with and use in structuring her life and activities

- feel that learning and discovery can be fun and interesting and that she has talents that she can use and share with others
- gain a new picture of what it means to be dyslexic
- do things and remember things in ways that work better and faster than the compulsive behaviours she has previously relied on

■ The follow-up programme

Once home with her box of tools the child who has completed the five-day Davis programme is really just at the beginning of the process that will lead to the full correction of her dyslexia. She will be practising using her newly acquired ability to be oriented when working with symbols and discovering the benefits of being oriented and able to control her orientation in situations where previously she might have become disoriented and confused.

The real work of correction, however, lies in removing all confusions from the words that have been triggering disorientation. There are just over 200 of these words that most dyslexics trigger on. By doing Symbol Mastery with these words – adding meanings to them in the form of pictures made in clay models – the sources of confusion are eliminated. This work should always be done in an easy and playful manner. The words are like little puzzles and you should make it clear to your child that making mistakes is fine and all part of the learning process. Working consistently with perhaps five words a week a child can have them all mastered within a year.

The support of parents is crucial for this phase of the correction. It requires persistence and patience and although the process does become easier there will be times when a child's flagging enthusiasm will need to be restored.

◼ Changes

Increased self-confidence

This part of the process of correction is perhaps the most rewarding for parents, although it can sometimes be overlooked if too much attention is paid to improvements in test scores or reading levels at school. A child's growth in self-confidence comes from having a picture of dyslexia that helps her make sense of what is going on and allows her to do something about it.

Giving up the old solution

By simply taking the tools she has learnt to use and applying them in her life, your child will gradually find ways of doing and learning things that work better than the compulsive solutions she has been using up to this point. The old solutions were, in fact, the true learning disability that your child was suffering from. This means that it is only when most of those old solutions are no longer being used that you can say your child has truly overcome her learning disability.

◼ Catching up at school

All the information and knowledge and skills that have not been acquired because of the learning disability have to be acquired once it is removed. What is often noted by children after completing a Davis treatment is how much they had actually learnt at school, despite their learning difficulties. The catching-up process therefore takes less time than if all the 'missed' information had to be learnt from scratch. What is also noticeable is that because a dyslexic child has often had to work so hard for years just to keep up with her class mates, once the obstructions to her learning are removed she is able to race ahead and often catches up with her peers in a shorter time than would be expected.

Symbol Mastery will help a dyslexic child to learn faster and more thoroughly. By being able to master fundamental concepts in a particular subject at school, she is able to think with those concepts much more effectively and creatively. The process is quite simple. It involves firstly getting a clear picture of the meaning of the concept or idea that needs to be mastered. That picture is then modelled in clay to create a real experience of the concept. The act of making an idea appear in a three-dimensional model makes that idea the child's own. Once an idea or meaning is mastered the child will never be able to forget it.

▓ Guidelines for parents

The wider perspective

All sorts of benefits and achievements and improvements will occur from the moment your child is able to control her disorientations, but the actual resolution of all the obstructions to learning is the technical end point of her training programme. As this process takes time to achieve, it is helpful to have this wider perspective on what is needed to correct the learning disability. This will be a very important part of your contribution to your child's training programme – to hold up the long-term point of view that she may lose when progress with Symbol Mastery slows down, as it may.

The following simple suggestions and guidelines have been found to be helpful for parents after their child has been through the training process described above.

1 Remember that the training your child receives in a Davis training programme should be seen as just the start to a whole process of change.

2 The more your child can understand and feel that it is her

responsibility to work with the tools obtained in the five-day training, the more likely it is that positive results will continue to show.

3 If it appears that progress in using the tools and mastering the confusing symbols is slowing down, look for any factors that might be interfering with the process, such as:

- Pressures in the classroom. A child's teacher or class mates may not know about or understand what she needs to help her correct her learning disabilities. The demands and pressures will still be there. Even though she now understands what she has to do, she may still feel unsure and nervous about using her newly acquired tools. She may even not want to talk about it for fear of being thought strange and different.
- Forgetting to use the tools. This is easily done in the rush and tumble of being back at school and trying to survive. It does take time and practice, especially for younger children, before they feel confident about using the tools and are assured of the results they can achieve.
- Resistance to the child's 'new status of independence'. She may know that she is now able to learn by herself, but because she always had your attention or special attention from a tutor she is afraid she will lose that attention if she starts to succeed at her work and become independent.

4 When a child goes through a Davis correction programme a great many internal processes are initiated that are not always visible on the surface. New feelings, new perceptions and ways of doing things are suddenly there in your child's life. What is needed most from parents is respect for what has been initiated and avoidance of any sort of pressure to move a child at a particular speed or in a particular direction through the processes of change.

5 It is known that a fundamental shift in awareness and understanding occurs as a result of doing the Davis Correction Programme. This shift begins a process of changes that sometimes takes months or even years to show its full effects. It is

from these slow, more subtle and internal processes that true growth and development in your child will come.

6 It helps, as said before, to see the Davis training as a process of removing obstructions to learning. Once these obstructions start to be removed your child can grow and develop natural abilities and talents. There is no way to predict the outcome of this growth.

7 Even if the weight of a child's learning disabilities starts to be lifted, another sort of pressure may mean that she is still unable to grow fully and express herself. The expectations, often unspoken, of parents and peers are just as powerful a restraining force as the compulsive old solutions. Be aware of your own expectations for your child and consciously create an environment where there is no pressure or stress. This is perhaps one of the most important forms of support you can give your child throughout this training programme.

8 Once the disability aspect begins to be removed, your child has a chance to be herself and express herself. Parents often exclaim excitedly that finally they have their real child back again. They have found the child they always knew was there but who was hidden behind the struggle with a learning disability.

9 It is very important that you feel you have the support of the counsellor who guided your child through the Davis programme. These counsellors are specially trained and understand what it requires from a child and from parents to fully make use of these tools. Each child will have her own particular way of taking and using the tools and there are many different scenarios for how the process of adaptation occurs.

Be sure to make use of the knowledge of your child's counsellor if you feel unsure at any point on how best to help her in the weeks and months after the initial training programme. It is very important to ensure that the natural momentum of removing the obstructions to learning is not stopped in a child by some simple question of confusion about how to use the tools. This obviously also applies to the teachers and tutors supporting your child who might want to know how best to help her at a particular stage in her development.

■ What you can do to support your child after completing a Davis programme

1 Congratulate her often on any improvement she has made, however small or insignificant it may seem to you at the beginning. What a child may see as a breakthrough in her process of change may go unnoticed by a parent unless this attitude of praise is always at the ready. On the other hand be careful not to be inappropriately enthusiastic – superficial praise for a dyslexic child is confusing. If you praise a child for something she does not feel particularly good about, she loses a point of reference to judge herself by. It can slow down the process of becoming sure and certain of her own abilities.

2 Don't be afraid to remind your child to use the tools and techniques she has learnt about at school and while doing homework. Do this by reminding her of her own choice and responsibility. Be careful not to use these tools as a way of manipulating and controlling or threatening your child.

3 Notice the moment a child is starting to demand too much of herself. Some children react to the pressures and expectations of school by pushing themselves too hard. Pressure prevents any child effectively using the tools she has learnt about. If she feels that she is a problem and is too much of a demand on her parents, guilt will also interfere with her ability to make use of and practise what she has learnt in her Davis training.

■ THE WAY FORWARD

The understanding of dyslexia given by Ron Davis' model can make a difference to how you see the future for your dyslexic child.

Dyslexia is not a permanent disability that will limit your child for the rest of her life. Your child now has the chance to assemble a box of tools to work with and remove her limitations and obstructions to learning. There is less need to try and predict or control the future for your child once she has these tools in her hands. Your child now has every chance to grow in self-confidence and independence. Your role will be to support your child in learning to enjoy her particular talents and ways of doing things, without concern.

■ CONCLUSION

The concepts and statements in this book can be justified and validated by you and your child only by testing them in your own experiences. Take the model for dyslexia that Ron Davis has provided and find out how they fit your own pictures. If they are useful and fit in a way that makes sense, you should certainly go ahead and make use of them. They are yours for the taking. Ron Davis offers these ideas freely to anyone who wants to try them out. They are yours as soon as you begin to apply them.

You will never know if you and your child can be helped by these ideas unless you test them out yourself. Because I know that many dyslexics have been able to enjoy relief from the burden of their learning disabilities, I can confidently offer these ideas to you and recommend you try them out.

There is an inherent satisfaction that comes whenever we get closer to reality and the truth of something. When we are able to get closer to understanding what is happening with a dyslexic child and are able to respond accordingly, remarkable changes can occur. Who your child really is will start to reveal itself.

I do hope this book will allow you and your child to be happy together in that simple satisfaction of knowing the truth about dyslexia.

Further Information on Dyslexia

The Orthodox Approach

The Internet is now the best and most inexpensive source of general information about orthodox approaches to dyslexia and also allows you to research any particular method of dyslexia treatment you may have heard about.

Because there is just so much information available it is good to have a plan before starting to do your search.

Here are some do's and don'ts when using the Internet:

- Don't try searching the Internet unless you are a little familiar with how to do this. It is best to ask someone else (usually your own children or someone younger than you!) who is familiar with the Internet and enjoys 'surfing' to do this for you.
- Don't do a general search under headings such as: 'dyslexia' or 'ADD' – you will get overwhelmed by all the information and will not know where to begin.
- Do be specific in what you are looking for – a particular name or method of treating dyslexia that you have heard about, or a particular set of symptoms that your child is suffering from.
- Do make use of Internet sites that are 'resource directories' about dyslexia. These are websites where a list of other websites about dyslexia is stored. They are often compiled by universities or associations for their own members but are made available to everyone. It means someone else has done the hard work of sorting through all the dyslexia websites for you.
- Do make use of 'discussion boards' on dyslexia. These are websites where you can follow discussions about a particular topic related to dyslexia, where you can ask questions about something you would like to know about, and share your interests or concerns. These discussion boards are an invaluable

source of information as they are mostly used by other people like yourself, who are looking for information or are sharing information about something they have found (either positive or negative). Discussion boards are also not controlled by any organisation that is promoting a particular product so, in general, you will find honest discussions about dyslexia by people who are very helpful, supportive and sympathetic. Often dyslexics themselves contribute to these discussion boards and their 'real-life' stories are the best source of information about whether a way of treating dyslexia does or does not work.

Two examples of these discussion boards are:

http://www.jiscmail.ac.uk/lists/dyslexia.html

http://www.dyslexiatalk.com/

The Davis Approach

The website about the Davis Approach (www.dyslexia.com) is the very best place to start finding out more information about all aspects of correcting dyslexia using the Davis methods.

You will find on this website names and addresses for Davis practitioners in many different countries around the world. These Davis facilitators can be contacted directly for more information and help. There is also a very useful resource section on the website, with many articles about learning differences and links to other sources of information.

Useful Addresses

Australia

SPELD
494 Brunswick St
North Fitzroy
Victoria, 3068
Tel.: +61 3 9489 4344
Fax: +61 3 9486 2437
Website: http://home.vicnet.net.au/~speld/

Ireland

ACLD (Association for Children and Adults with Learning Disabilities)
Head Office
Suffolk Chambers
1 Suffolk Street
Dublin 2
Tel.: 01 6790276
Fax: 01 6790273
E-mail: acld@iol.ie
Website: http://www.iol. ie/~acld/

Northern Ireland Dyslexia Association
17a Upper Newtownards Road
Belfast BT4 3HT
Tel.: 028 9065 9212
E-mail: help@nida.org.uk
Website: http://www.nida.org.uk/

New Zealand

SPELD
PO Box 27112
Wellington
E-mail: speldauckland@clear.net.nz
Website: http://www.speld.org.nz/

Scotland

The Scottish Dyslexia Association (SDA)
Stirling Business Centre
Wellgreen
Stirling FK8 2DZ
Tel.: 01786 446650
Fax: 01786 471235
Website: http://www.dyslexia.scotland.dial.pipex.com/

UK

Adult Dyslexia Organisation
336 Brixton Rd
London SW9 7AA
Tel.: 020 7924 9559
Website: http://www.futurenet.com/charity/ado/

The British Dyslexia Association
98 London Road
Reading
Berkshire RG1 5AU
Tel.: 0118 966 8271

The Dyslexia Institute
133 Gresham Rd
Staines
Middlesex TW18 2AJ
Tel.: 01784 463851

The Hornsby International Dyslexia Centre
Wye St
London SW11 2HB
Tel.: 020 7223 1144

The Sound Learning Centre
12 The Rise
London N13 5LE
Tel.: 020 8882 1060

USA

The International Dyslexia Association
8600 LaSalle Road
Chester Building
Suite 382
Baltimore, MD 21286-2044
Tel.: 410 296 0232
Fax: 410 321 5069
Website: http://www.interdys.org/

Learning Disabilities Association of America
4156 Library Road
Pittsburgh, PA 15234-1349
Tel.: 412 341 1515
Fax: 412 344 0224
E-mail: info@ldaamerica.org/
Website: http://www.ldanatl.org/

National Center for Learning Disabilities
381 Park Avenue South
Suite 1401
New York, NY 10016
Tel.: 212 545 7510
Tel.: (Toll-Free): 888 575 7373
Fax: 212 545 9665
Website: http://www.ncld.org/

Slingerland Institute
One Bellevue Center
411 108th. Ave. NE
Bellevue, WA 98004
Tel.: 425 453 1190
Fax.: 425 635 7762
E-mail: mail@slingerland.org
Website: http://www.slingerland.org/

CHADD (Children and Adults with Attention-Deficit Disorder)
8181 Professional Place
Suite 201

Landover, MD 20785
Tel.: 301 306 7070
Tel.: (Toll-Free): 800 233 4050
Fax: 301 306 7090
E-mail: national@chadd.org
Website: http://www.chadd.org/

THE DAVIS APPROACH

Germany

DDA Deutschland
Conventstr. 14
D-22089 Hamburg
Tel.: +49 040 25 17 86 22
Fax: +49 040 25 17 8624
E-mail: germany@dyslexia.com
Website: http://www.dyslexia.de

Mexico

DDA Mexico
Contact: Olga Zambrano de Carrillo Privada Fuentes
110 Col Santa Engracia Garza Garcia
Monterrey N.L.
Tel.: 8 335 94 35
Fax: 8 356 83 89
E-mail: puertadeletras@infosel.net.mx
Website: http://www.dyslexia.com/mexico/

The Netherlands

DDA-Nederland
Kerkweg 38a
6105 CG Maria Hoop
Tel.: +31 0475 301 277
Fax: +31 0475 301 381
E-mail: holland@dyslexia.com

Switzerland

DDA–CH
Freie Strasse 81
CH 4001 Basel
Tel.: +41 61 273 81 85
Fax: +41 61 272 42 41
E-mail: switzerland@dyslexia.com
Website: http://www.dda.ch

UK

DDA–UK
PO Box 40
Winchester SO22 6ZH
Tel.: +44 01962 820005
Fax: +44 01962 820006
E-mail: uk@dyslexia.com

USA

Davis Dyslexia Association International
1601 Bayshore Highway
Suite 245
Burlingame, CA 94010
Tel.: 650 692 7141
Fax: 650 692 7075
E-mail: ddai@dyslexia.com
Website: http://www.dyslexia.com/ddai.htm

Index